THE
MYTH OF
SANITY

THE
MYTH OF
SANITY

Divided

Consciousness

and

the Promise of

Awareness

MARTHA STOUT

VIKING

VIKING
Published by the Penguin Group
Penguin Putnam Inc., 375 Hudson Street, New York, New York 10014, U.S.A.
Penguin Books Ltd, 27 Wrights Lane, London W8 5TZ, England
Penguin Books Australia Ltd, Ringwood, Victoria, Australia
Penguin Books Canada Ltd, 10 Alcorn Avenue, Toronto, Ontario, Canada M4V 3B2
Penguin Books (N.Z.) Ltd, 182–190 Wairau Road, Auckland 10, New Zealand

Penguin Books Ltd, Registered Offices:
Harmondsworth, Middlesex, England

First published in 2001 by Viking Penguin,
a member of Penguin Putnam Inc.

10   9   8   7   6   5   4   3   2   1

LIBRARY OF CONGRESS CATALOGING IN PUBLICATION DATA

Stout, Martha.
    The myth of sanity : divided consciousness and the promise of awareness / Martha Stout.
    p.   cm.
    Includes bibliographical references and index.
    ISBN 0–670–89475–3
    1. Dissociative disorders.   2. Adult child abuse victims.   3. Post-traumatic stress
disorder.   I. Title.

RC553.D5 S76 2001
616.85'23—dc21   00–043994

This book is printed on acid-free paper. ∞

Printed in the United States of America
Set in Janson Text
Designed by Nancy Resnick

Written, with love and gratitude,
for my mother and father

Eva Deaton Stout
and
Adrian Phillip Stout

With our thoughts, we make the world.

—Buddha

The idea of earning a doctoral degree, which later turned into a lifelong career in the psychology of trauma, was first suggested to me by my father's mother, who was born a quarter of a century before women had the right to vote, in the backwoods of North Carolina. She was a woman of great faith and strength—with more than a few radical opinions for her time—and she endured much during her nearly eighty years on this earth. Yet when the end came, she willingly relinquished her life.

To be more precise, I could say that my grandmother willed her own death. Lying in a hospital bed, being attended for minor cardiac difficulties in a heart relatively strong for a woman her age, she informed her nurse one night, simply, that she would go to God before morning. The nurse, I am told, kindly reassured her she was not so ill as all that, and that she should not think such thoughts. My grandmother died that night, inexplicably, of congestive heart failure.

When she died, I was a junior in college, and it was there that I learned the implications of congestive heart failure. Voodoo victims die that way, victims of their own strength of belief, and other mammals, swimming against the tide for too long, let death come, and die of exploding hearts, before the water has a chance to drown them. Having decided it is time, one simply dies.

As a therapist, I see trauma survivors, and in the course of my profession I have heard the life stories of dozens and hundreds of people who have survived childhood and adult circumstances of unrelenting horror. The vague whisper I heard through knowing my grandmother, that life was not always so gentle as my childhood, has become a frank cacophony of excruciating human histories.

And now it is my trauma patients who seem the oldest souls in the world, though some of them are quite young people. They are proud human spirits who seem ancient and ageless at the same time. Over the years, I have seen brighter passions in their eyes than in the eyes of any priest or guru. I have heard more wisdom from their mouths than I have read in any book. And, ironically I suppose, I have at times experienced a more profound and centered stillness in their presence than in the company of people whose histories and memories have been far less scarred.

My patients come from both genders, and all walks of life. Some are simple. Others possess intellects as brilliant and faceted as diamonds. Most are somewhere in between. They come to my office bearing a wide variety of diagnoses currently in medical vogue: depression, manic-depressive disorder, panic disorder, anorexia nervosa, alcoholism, borderline personality disorder, paranoia. Their stories are seemingly diverse. Some have survived earthquakes. One, when she was two years old, watched from inside the basket someone had hidden her in, as her Cambodian parents and nine sisters and brothers were shot to death by invading soldiers. Many others have survived chronic childhood incest. And still others are adult survivors of other kinds of childhood-long abuse, physical and psychological.

But I have learned that they all have one thing in common. Underlying the various forms of heartrending pain and diverse complaints with which they come to therapy is the same fundamental question—*Shall I choose to die, or shall I choose to live?* They come to therapy to help themselves answer that question, and I will get nowhere if I try to answer the question for them, or even delay its consideration. The rest of therapy never begins for a survivor of trauma until that ruthlessly basic question has been answered.

I cannot resolve the life-or-death question for my patients, and I should confess that I do not even approach the practice of psychotherapy with the premise about suicide that is widely held to be self-evident. Many say it is necessarily our job to insure that no individual be allowed to carry out a decision to die, that it is our job to prevent this no matter what the measure taken to prevent it, be that measure manipulative, legal, even legally violent. But I do not believe, nor can I be persuaded, that some form of psychological distortion underlies absolutely all acts of suicide. I do believe that, at least in some cases, a decision to die could be just that, a decision. This seems obvious and simple enough to me.

And I have come to accept that a person can consciously or unconsciously terminate biological existence in a variety of ways, most of them not preventable by me or anyone else, regardless of ideology. For example, my grandmother decided to die when she did, or that is my belief anyway. Having known Fleeta Florence Stout, I am not surprised she was capable of that. What impresses me is that for eighty years she chose to live—not just to not die, but to live—passionately, consciously, full of faith, despite all the hardships and sorrows of her time here.

Moreover, I have learned through my work that most people need look back only a generation or two, if at all, to find survivors in their own families—individuals who have somehow found the strength and the faith to go on living—and that the nearness of trauma, and of survival's impossible choices, has powerful and unexplored implications for the human family as a whole.

The survivors I see in my practice have known undistilled fear, have seen how nakedly terrifying life can be, and in many cases have seen how starkly ugly their fellow human beings can be. Listening to their stories, no one at all could be surprised that they consider the possibility of not going on. In a struggle with the power of their past experiences, even the biological imperative to survive is puny.

No. Their choosing to die would not be surprising. What is so extraordinary about these people is that they choose to live—not just to not die, not just to survive, but to live.

Why this choice gets made, and how it gets put into practice, are two of the most interesting personal, psychological, and philosophical questions I can conceive of. And one of the greatest privileges of my life has been to know the people who are my patients, to be able to sit with them, to be a part of their lives for a while, and with grateful and undisguised self-interest, to *listen*. For I have become convinced that these courageous people, in winning their struggles, must learn things about genuine living, and about genuine sanity, that the rest of us have never even imagined.

ACKNOWLEDGMENTS

First, I would like to thank my friend and brilliant colleague, Carol Kauffman, on whose patio this book was invented one sunny Memorial Day, and who has seen me all the way through to the end. Without cease and without complaint, she has provided motivation, note-perfect advice, and the priceless favor of her expert commentary. And I would like to thank (a million times thank!) my heaven-sent agent, Susan Lee Cohen, whose wisdom, balance, and loveliness of spirit inaugurated the project and kept it alive.

Thanks to the gifted Beena Kamlani, for her integrity, for her beautiful and meticulous editing, and for that uncanny guiding voice in my head, and to Carole DeSanti, for recognizing the manuscript in the first place, and for her relentless advocacy of the book at Viking. My gratitude also to Alexandra Babanskyj, and to Jaime Wolf.

For having helped me in their various crucial ways to complete the book, I would like to thank Jane Delgado (an inspiration even now), Paul Horovitz, Deborah Horvitz, Judith Jordan, Howard Kielley, Martin Seligman, David Stein, and Len Thomas.

And I would like to thank my patients, every single one of them.

I thank my brother and my beloved friend, Steve Stout, for his matchless intellect and heart, and all the splendid conversations of a lifetime. I thank Eva Deaton Stout and Adrian Phillip Stout, who are what all parents should be in a perfect world. And, of course, I would like to express my endless gratitude to my exquisite daughter, Amanda, for being Amanda.

CONTENTS

Preface   *ix*

Acknowledgments   *xiii*

PART ONE: DISSOCIATION   1

Chapter One: Old Souls   3

Chapter Two: When I Woke Up Tuesday Morning,
      It Was Friday   15

PART TWO: THE SHELL-SHOCKED SPECIES   45

Chapter Three: Duck and Cover   47

Chapter Four: Pieces of Me   67

Chapter Five: The Human Condition   104

PART THREE: SPLIT IDENTITY   133

Chapter Six: Replaced   135

Chapter Seven: Switchers   159

PART FOUR: SANITY   199

Chapter Eight: Why Parker Was Parker   201

Chapter Nine: As it Should Be   223

Notes   *237*

Index   *245*

AUTHOR'S NOTE

With the exception of the passages concerning my own family history, the descriptions in *The Myth of Sanity* do not identify individuals. At the very heart of psychotherapy is the precept of confidentiality, and I have taken the most exacting measures to preserve the privacy of all real persons. All names are fictitious, and all other recognizable features have been changed.

Some individuals who appear in the book willingly gave their consent to be anonymously portrayed. In these cases, no information has been included that might in any way identify them. Otherwise, the people, events, and conversations presented here are composite in nature; that is to say, each case represents a great many individuals whose characteristics and experiences have been adopted conceptually, carefully altered in their specifics, and combined to form an illustrative character. Any resemblance of such a composite character to any actual person is entirely coincidental.

THE
MYTH OF
SANITY

DISSOCIATION

CHAPTER ONE

Old Souls

*How does one kill fear, I wonder? How do you shoot a
spectre through the heart, slash off its spectral head, take
it by the spectral throat?*

—Joseph Conrad

We are all a little crazy.

In listening to my patients tell me thousands of stories about the past, as they try to find some peace in the present, I have learned this beyond the shadow of a doubt. Rather than behaving sanely, rather than being in touch with our present realities, we human beings—all of us, myself included—are too often simply run by losses and hardships long gone by, and by our stockpiled fears. Our collective history, our individual lives, our very minds, bear unmistakable testimony.

Instead of receding harmlessly into the past, the darkest, most frightening events of childhood and adolescence gain power and authority as we grow older. The memory of these events causes us to depart from ourselves, psychologically speaking, or to separate one part of our awareness from the others. What we conceive of as an unbroken thread of consciousness is instead quite often a train of discontinuous fragments. Our awareness is divided. And much more commonly than we know, even our personalities are fragmented—disorganized team efforts trying to cope with the past—rather than the sane, unified wholes we anticipate in ourselves and in other people.

Is this our unalterable destiny as human beings, or are there some authentic solutions?

In my capacity as a therapist for trauma survivors, I have spent twenty years listening to people's stories, to the recounting of experiences so nightmarish, so abusive, and so abhorrent that one might well wish never to have known about them. Then it has been my privilege to know these same people as they recovered from their past experiences, and learned how to live in the present. And I believe that their stories contain meaningful lessons in how to leave behind some of our own long-ago terrors. There are possible solutions that come as gifts to the rest of us from the old souls, the exceptional survivors.

I began my practice by specializing in the treatment of people suffering from medically threatening anorexia and intractable depressive disorders. Also, for better or not, I developed a professional reputation as someone willing to take on individuals who were on the edge, patients whose potential for suicide or other self-destructive behavior had placed them at high risk. Gradually, I began to notice that, too consistently to be ignored, most of the people I was treating were survivors of extreme psychological trauma, and that their symptoms tended to match the phenomenon of post-traumatic stress disorder just as closely as the more traditional diagnoses.

Sometimes I think of my lifework as overall lessons learned, themes, discoveries. But much more instructively and frequently, I think in terms of the individual human beings whom my profession has brought to me. On a certain level, I feel tied to many of these people with a knot so tight that I readily understand the appeal of notions such as fate, or even karma.

I believe I was drawn to them for their fire. The honest, purposeful self-examination of a traumatized life creates a heat so exquisite that it burns away the usual appeasements, self-deceptions, and defenses. "What is the meaning of this life?" becomes a very personal question, and demands an answer. Some of the people I have known have burned so fiercely that they have gone all-stop, have quit their jobs, even endured temporary poverty, because answering the question consumed more energy than can reasonably be generated by a solitary individual. There is something electric in the eyes, a little wild.

But paradoxically—and yet, I think, for all the same reasons—these same people often reveal an irresistible sense of humor, an ironic angle on life that has dispensed with the polite and the guarded, and that tends to get right to the core of things. And so, though it may sound odd, when I am with my patients, I laugh out loud a lot.

Many trauma patients are detached and objective when they speak of extraordinary events, such as the particulars of failed suicide attempts, that most other people, if they speak of such matters at all, tend to cushion with lengthy introductions and euphemisms. As I listen to the telling of a personal history, more often than overt "symptoms," it is just such Faulkneresque understatement of the sometimes macabre, along with the burning light in the eyes, and the cunning humor, that makes me begin to suspect extreme trauma in the individual's history.

As a psychologist, and as a human being, I am impressed with the irony that these severely traumatized patients, people who have been through living nightmares, people who might blamelessly choose death, often emerge from successful treatment by constructing lives for themselves that are freer than most ordinary lives from what Sigmund Freud, a century ago, labeled as "everyday misery." They become true keepers of the faith and are the most passionately alive people I know.

Or maybe it is more necessity than irony. I have been told more than once by the survivors of trauma that it would not be worth the struggle merely to go on surviving. And that is exactly what most of the rest of us do: we do not choose to die, or to live; we go on surviving. We do not choose nonexistence; nor do we choose complete awareness. We slog on, in a kind of foggy cognitive middle-land we call sane, a place where we almost never acknowledge the haze.

Over the years, what my trauma patients have taught me is that this compromise with reality and its traumas is simply not sanity at all. It is a form of madness, and it befuddles our existence. We lose parts of our thoughts in the present, we sabotage the closeness and comfort in our relationships, and we misplace important pieces of ourselves.

All of us are exposed to some amount of psychological trauma at some point in our lives, and yet most of us are unaware of the misty spaces in our brains left there by traumatic experience, since for the most part we experience them only indirectly. Seldom do we ponder the traumatic events in our own lives, let alone the fright-ening hardships and life-or-death struggles that were the daily lot of people as close to us, in terms of time, as our great-grandmothers, or even our grandmothers.

But we do feel crazy, and a little silly, when from time to time we cannot remember a simple thing we ought to be able to remember. ("Early-onset Alzheimer's," people will joke—neither morbidly nor quite lightheartedly.)

And we feel our insanity, and sometimes a near-frantic sense of being out of control of our lives, in the misunderstandings and rifts in our most cherished relationships, in the same emotionally mud-dled arguments that go on for years and years. The conflicts never quite kill the love that we feel, but they never quite end either. And as a society, we feel incompetent, and sinkingly helpless, when we re-flect upon the greater-than-half failure rate of marriages in general.

Too many of us walk on eggshells around our life partners, the-oretically the very people whom we should know the best. We do this because we are never certain when that lover or that spouse is going to become aggrieved, or fall silent, or fly into an impenetrable rage at something that happens, or at something we have said, and become a distant stranger, a different person altogether whom, in all honesty, we do not know at all.

Or we look at our parents as they grow older, and seeing that time is running out, we long to be closer to them, to know them as friends. But when we actually try to think about accomplishing this, our thoughts skitter away from us like frightened deer from an open meadow, and in the next moment our minds are elsewhere—anywhere else—the rising price of gasoline, a memo at work, a spot on the carpet.

Many of us find it difficult, and sometimes impossible, to stay in one "mode," to be constant and recognizable, even to ourselves. One of the most universal examples of this is the experience of returning "home" to one's parents. After a family visit, the commonest revelation, sometimes private and sometimes voiced aloud to friends, is "I turn into a different person. I can't help it. I just do. All of a sudden I'm thirteen again." We are completely grown up and may even consider ourselves to be rather sophisticated. We understand how we ought to act, know what we want to say to our mothers and our fathers. We have plans. But when we get there, we cannot follow through—because suddenly we are not really there. Needy, out-of-control children have taken over our bodies, and are acting in our stead. And we are helpless to get our "real" selves back until well after we have departed from our "homes" once again.

Perhaps worst of all, as time passes we often feel that we are growing benumbed, that we have lost *something*—some element of vitality that used to be there. Without talking about this very much with one another, we grow nostalgic for our own selves. We try to remember the exuberance, and even the joy, we used to feel in things. And we cannot. Mysteriously, and before we realize what is happening, our lives are transfigured from places of imagination and hope into to-do lists, into day after day of just getting through it. Often we are able to envision only a long road of exhausting hurdles, that leads to somewhere we are no longer at all certain we even want to go. Instead of having dreams, we merely protect ourselves. We expend our brief and precious life force in the practice of damage control.

And all because of traumatic events that occurred in the long-ago past, that *ended* in the long-ago past, and that, in actuality, threaten us with no present danger whatsoever. How does this happen? How do childhood and adolescent terrors that should have been over years ago manage to live on and make us crazy, and alienated from ourselves, in the present?

The answer, paradoxically, lies in a perfectly normal function of the mind known as *dissociation*, which is the universal human reaction to extreme fear or pain. In traumatic situations, dissociation mercifully allows us to disconnect emotional content—the feeling part of our "selves"—from our conscious awareness. Disconnected from our feelings in this way, we stand a better chance of surviving the ordeal, of doing what we have to do, of getting through a critical moment in which our emotions would only be in the way. Dissociation causes a person to view an ongoing traumatic event almost as if she were a spectator, and this separation of emotion from thought and action, the spectator's perspective, may well prevent her from being utterly overwhelmed on the spot.

A moderate dissociative reaction—after a car crash, for example—is typically expressed as, "I felt as if I were just *watching* myself go through it. I wasn't even scared."

Dissociation during trauma is extremely adaptive; it is a survival function. The problem comes later—for long after the ordeal is over, the tendency to be disconnected from our selves may remain. Our old terrors train us to be dissociative, to feel safe by taking little psychological vacations from reality when it is too frightening or painful. But later, these mental vacations may come upon us even when we do not need them, or want them—or recognize them. For no conspicuous reason, we depart from ourselves, and people we care about depart from themselves, and these unrecognized psychological absences play havoc with our lives and our loves.

Unsurprisingly, survivors of extreme psychological trauma have extreme dissociative reactions, and listening to my trauma patients has allowed me to understand not only dissociation itself, but also the ways in which people may overcome the numbing and unwanted outcomes of dissociative experience. Listening to my patients, I have come to believe in the possibility, for all of us, of staying in touch with reality, of becoming truly sane. If these people can learn to remain present with the reality of their memories, if they can make a commitment to live their lives consciously and meaningfully, so can we.

For the mental universe of the extreme trauma survivor is so full of violence and violation, natural demons and unnatural acts, that one wonders—I wonder every day—how such people find the courage to decide to go on living. It is a place where trusting someone is not an option, and where the genius of one's own imagination becomes an inescapable stalker. In such a landscape, whenever the inhabitant becomes so bone-weary that she lets down her guard a little, another memory cabinet door swings open to reveal precisely the thing that she cannot endure. This thing is different for each person, but always hovers at the outside limit of terror. Letting down her guard is at once what she most achingly desires and what she most vigilantly avoids. It is a universe of fear and exhaustion—especially exhaustion—and people will try almost anything, however irrational, to make it stop.

As a therapist for survivors, I routinely witness extremes of human behavior for which neither my personal history nor my formal education in psychology could have prepared me even minimally. Survivors are often what the uncompassionate vocabulary of psychiatric hospitals refers to as "cutters." This means that unrecovered survivors of early trauma often inflict bloody injuries upon themselves—deep cuts and third-degree burns—not necessarily with death as a goal, but rather out of some compelling sense that the injuries themselves are necessary. For the most part, these acts of self-abuse are carried out methodically and repetitively, and with a chilling awareness of the practicalities of injury. Some of my patients learn to bandage themselves as well as any nurse could, and when a trip to the emergency room is required, they have already prepared a socially acceptable answer to "How did this happen to you?" and offer it calmly when asked.

The doctors believe the story, and no one recognizes the desperate situation of the person into whose arm the stitches are going.

In a seeming contradiction to self-injury, prior to recovery some trauma survivors study, buy, and stockpile weapons against outside threats. Sometimes a certain special weapon will be concealed and carried with the person, as routinely as someone else might wear a wristwatch. The concealed mace or knife or gun seems to be a defense against a horrible, nameless danger that never materializes but is constantly expected, a testimony to the monstrous threat the individual knew in the past, and was unable to defend herself against. Whether or not a weapon could have prevented the original trauma does not seem to be important. What is important is a kind of material insurance that one is not nakedly helpless like before.

The busy professional person no one would ever suspect may very well make a confession in therapy, and show me the unused but studiously maintained knife she hides inside her boot.

The forms of extreme behavior can be dramatic, or they can be obscure and progressive. In my experience, the profoundest cases of anorexia nervosa (self-starvation syndrome) are always trauma survivors, usually survivors of sexual abuse. Like the despairing victims of voodoo, those afflicted with profound anorexia also sometimes die of congestive heart failure, but by a slower mechanism. This was the case with Marcie, a patient who recently entered treatment with me after having technically died twice, and having been twice revived by the physicians.

This is what happens when the cause is anorexia: in cases of advanced starvation, the body cannot get enough protein to survive. It must begin to feed upon its own internal sources of protein, for example, the muscle tissue of the heart. When the heart has been sufficiently damaged, it can no longer pump blood well enough, and congestive heart failure results.

My new patient Marcie starved herself to death when she was twenty. She wonders why she did not see bright lights and hear the angels. But more than that, she wonders why the doctors saved her.

"Do you like my new shoes?" she asks me now. "I got them for four dollars and ninety-eight cents in Harvard Square. I haven't had new shoes in three years."

"Why, Marcie?" I ask.

"I don't like to have so many things for myself, you know? Some people can have lots of things, but it just makes me nervous, you know? I don't need too many things for me."

"I'm glad you bought the shoes."

"Do you really like them?"

"They're very pretty, Marcie."

Marcie is my height, five feet five inches tall, but when she first arrived at the hospital in Boston, after her "deaths" in a New York hospital, she weighed sixty-eight pounds, a fetus in fetal position in a psychiatric seclusion room. Today, two years later, she weighs 115 pounds—according to the charts, a reasonable weight. But pale, troubled, looking out from behind her large round glasses, and feeling that she is fifty pounds overweight, she is still more spirit than body.

No more seclusion room now. Marcie takes the Red Line, and the Green Line. To Harvard Square. To Boston, to see me. To see *The Tin Drum.*

Why why why why? she asks.

Why are people like that? Why do people have to be like that? She asks me, over and over. Why? She asks Günter Grass.

Why?

Oh yes, survivors' hearts and histories are torn and scarred, in all the ways one would expect, and in a multitude of ways one could never imagine. And by now I could own a macabre collection of

potential suicide instruments—nooses, pills, hypodermic nee-
dles—given up to me by survivors, often quite ceremoniously, as
they begin to recover.

But after recovery, after they have chosen to live, these same
people often truly live—passionately, in a way many other people
never achieve. Survivors embody extremes of human experience,
such that everyday misery is a near-stranger to them. At first, their
pain is much worse than our everyday misery, by a factor so large that
it would be difficult for most to conceive of it. And then later, after recovery, everyday misery is simply unacceptable. Life must be a pas-
sionate, conscious journey, or it is just not worth the survival effort.

In the context of their own personal experience, and their struggle to come to terms with it, survivors inevitably address certain
questions. Does anyone ever truly care about anyone else? Is love
just a word? On this planet, is it possible to be in control of anything? Is it all right not to be in control? Does human life, in its
pain and vulnerability, contain something that makes it worth-
while? And these questions are not addressed philosophically, from
the relatively detached stance the rest of us may enjoy at times, but
rather from a position of intense and consumingly personal rele-
vancy every day.

Eventually, the trauma survivors I see glean their own answers
to some of the most fundamental human questions. And the be-
liefs, strategies, and personal values they come to live by are fascinating, a school for human life. Perhaps most instructive of all is
the recovered trauma survivor's intimate relationship with what is
for many people the most distant of philosophical concepts: awareness of the truth. That awareness is life-giving, that dissociation
and numbness are lethal, is a lesson the recovered survivor has
learned down to his or her bones. It is the lesson that sparks the
missionary's glint. It restores faith, and makes living a workable
choice. And though the turnabout may seem ironic, this lesson is
precisely the one that many of us have not learned deeply enough
to make genuine living possible. Perhaps, like grandchildren, we
can learn it from the old souls, from the survivors.

I myself understand whatever I do about these things because I have had the rare privilege of listening to the people who are my patients. I listen, for example, to Marcie, she who was twice dead and twice revived by the doctors, she who is now twenty-two years old and also as old as the world. If Marcie chooses to live, it seems to me that what she will have to say about human life is prophecy, fascinating and true as any the race will ever receive.

Marcie is from Albany, New York, where the fantastical pink granite State Capitol stands at the head of State Street. In Marcie's house in Albany, she was repeatedly beaten and raped by her crazy father and her crazier older brother, until she was old enough to get out.

Marcie's voice is flat when she speaks of Albany.

I have already heard that her father abused both his children, and that her brother, in his turn, abused Marcie. Rape handed down from father to son. I have already heard that Marcie's helplessly depressed mother would rock in her rocking chair for hours at a time, intoning "Oh no, oh no," over and over to no one in particular. On the day Marcie's father finally abandoned the family, that was what her mother was doing. I have heard that Marcie's brother eventually received a diagnosis of schizophrenia, in an Albany hospital I cannot contact because Marcie cannot remember its name.

"I remember once I locked myself in my mother's room and called the police. When the police came, my brother went to the door and told them everything was fine. They went away. I climbed out the window and hid for a long, long time. It was dark when I came back. I knew how mad they'd be."

I look up at the abstract painting that hangs behind Marcie's chair in my office, and in my own mind I repeat Marcie's question—why? And will you decide to stay with us anyway, Marcie? I silently ask her. Will you choose to continue your life, or will you keep trying to end it?

She looks over at me in my chair, and as if reading my mind she asks, "What do people do with all that time? I mean, people other than me. They must do something. All those nights and weekends for years and years. I can't even imagine what I'm going to do with all that time. Don't people get awfully tired after a while? I mean, won't I get awfully tired? And is there something that makes it okay in the end? Is there something that makes it worth it, being so tired, going through all this?"

I don't know, Marcie, I think to myself. One day you will walk in here and you will tell me.

CHAPTER TWO

When I Woke Up Tuesday Morning, It Was Friday

> *"The horror of that moment," the King went on,*
> *"I shall never, never forget!"*
> *"You will, though," the Queen said, "if you don't*
> *make a memorandum of it."*
>
> —Lewis Carroll

I magine that you are in your house—no—you are *locked* in your house, cannot get out. It is the dead of winter. The drifted snow is higher than your windows, blocking the light of both moon and sun. Around the house, the wind moans, night and day.

Now imagine that even though you have plenty of electric lights, and perfectly good central heating, you are almost always in the dark and quite cold, because something is wrong with the old-fashioned fuse box in the basement. Inside this cobwebbed, innocuous-looking box, the fuses keep burning out, and on account of this small malfunction, all the power in the house repeatedly fails. You have replaced so many melted fuses that now your little bag of new ones is empty; there are no more. You sigh in frustration, and regard your frozen breath in the light of the flashlight. Your house, which could be so cozy, is tomblike instead.

In all probability, there is something quirky in the antiquated fuse box; it has developed some kind of needless hair trigger, and is not really reacting to any dangerous electrical overload at all. Should you get some pennies out of your pocket, and use them to replace the burned-out fuses? That would solve the power-outage problem. No more shorts, not with copper coins in there. Using coins would scuttle the safeguard function of the fuse box, but the need for a safeguard right now is questionable, and the box is keeping you cold and in the dark for no good reason. Well, probably for no good reason.

On the other hand, what if the wiring in the house really is overloaded somehow? A fire could result, probably will result eventually. If you do not find the fire soon enough, if you cannot manage to put the fire out, the whole house could go up, with you trapped inside. You know that death by burning is hideous. You know also that your mind is playing tricks, but thinking about fire, you almost imagine there is smoke in your nostrils right now.

So, do you go back upstairs and sit endlessly in a dark living room, defeated, numb from the cold, though you have buried yourself under every blanket in the house? No light to read by, no music, just the wail and rattle of the icy wind outside? Or, in an attempt to feel more human, do you make things warm and comfortable? Is it wise to gamble with calamity and howling pain? If you turn the power back on, will you not smell nonexistent smoke every moment you are awake? And will you not have far too many of these waking moments, for how will you ever risk going to sleep?

Do you sabotage the fuse box?

I believe that most of us cannot know what we would do, trapped in a situation that required such a seemingly no-win decision. But I do know that anyone wanting to recover from psychological trauma must face just this kind of dilemma, made yet more harrowing because her circumstance is not anything so rescuable as being locked in a house, but rather involves a solitary, unlockable confinement inside the limits of her own mind. The person who suffers from a severe trauma disorder must decide between surviving in a barely sublethal misery of numbness and frustration, and taking a chance that may well bring her a better life, but that feels like stupidly issuing an open invitation to the unspeakable horror that waits to consume her alive. And in the manner of the true hero, she must choose to take the risk.

For trauma changes the brain itself. Like the outdated fuse box, the psychologically traumatized brain houses inscrutable eccentricities that cause it to overreact—or more precisely, *mis*react—to the current realities of life. These neurological misreactions become established because trauma has a profound effect upon the secretion of stress-responsive neurohormones such as norepinephrine, and thus an effect upon various areas of the brain involved in memory, particularly the amygdala and the hippocampus.

The amygdala receives sensory information from the five senses, via the thalamus, attaches emotional significance to the input, and then passes along this emotional "evaluation" to the hippocampus. In accordance with the amygdala's "evaluation" of importance, the hippocampus is activated to a greater or lesser degree, and functions to organize the new input, and to integrate it with already existing information about similar sensory events. Under a normal range of conditions, this system works efficiently to consolidate memories according to their emotional priority. However, at the extreme upper end of hormonal stimulation, as in traumatic situations, a breakdown occurs. Overwhelming emotional significance registered by the amygdala actually leads to a *decrease in hippocampal activation*, such that some of the traumatic input is not usefully organized by the hippocampus, or integrated with other memories. The result is that portions of traumatic memory are stored not as parts of a unified whole, but as isolated sensory images and bodily sensations that are not localized in time or even in situation, or integrated with other events.

To make matters still more complex, exposure to trauma may

temporarily shut down Broca's area, the region of the left hemi-sphere of the brain that translates experience into language, the means by which we most often relate our experience to others, and even to ourselves.

A growing body of research indicates that in these ways the brain lays down traumatic memories differently from the way it records regular memories. Regular memories are formed through adequate hippocampal and cortical input, are integrated as com-prehensible wholes, and are subject to meaning-modification by future events, and through language. In contrast, traumatic mem-ories include chaotic fragments that are sealed off from modula-tion by subsequent experience. Such memory fragments are wordless, placeless, and eternal, and long after the original trauma has receded into the past, the brain's record of it may consist only of isolated and thoroughly anonymous bits of emotion, image, and sensation that ring through the individual like a broken alarm.

Worse yet, later in the individual's life, in situations that are vaguely similar to the trauma—perhaps merely because they are startling, anxiety-provoking, or emotionally arousing—amygdala-mediated memory traces are accessed more readily than are the more complete, less shrill memories that have been integrated and modified by the hippocampus and the cerebral cortex. Even though unified and updated memories would be more judicious in the present, the amygdala memories are more accessible, and so trauma may be "remembered" at inappropriate times, when there is no hazard worthy of such alarm. In reaction to relatively trivial stresses, the person traumatized long ago may truly *feel* that danger is imminent again, be assailed full-force by the emotions, bodily sensations, and perhaps even the images, sounds, smells that once accompanied great threat.

Here is an illustration from everyday life. A woman named Bev-erly reads a morning newspaper while she sits at a quiet suburban depot and waits for a train. The article, concerning an outrageous local scandal, intrigues her so much that for a few minutes she for-gets where she is. Suddenly, there is an earsplitting blast from the train as it signals its arrival. Beverly is painfully startled by the noise; her head snaps up, and she catches her breath. She is amazed that she could have been so lacking in vigilance and relaxed in public. Her heart pounds, and in the instant required to fold the newspaper, she is ambushed by bodily feelings and even a smell that have nothing whatever to do with the depot on this uneventful morning. If she could identify the smell, which she never will, she would call it "chlorine." She feels a sudden rigidity in her chest, as if her lungs had just turned to stone, and has an almost overpowering impulse to get out of there, to run.

In a heartbeat, the present is perceptually and emotionally the past. These fragments of sensation and emotion are the amygdala-mediated memories of an afternoon three decades before, in Beverly's tenth summer, when, walking home from the public swimming pool, she saw her younger sister skip into the street and meet an immediate death in front of a speeding car. At this moment, thirty years later, Beverly *feels* that way again.

Her sensations and feelings are not labeled as belonging to memories of the horrible accident. In fact, they are not labeled as anything at all, because they have always been completely without language. They belong to no narrative, no place or time, no story she can tell about her life; they are free-form and ineffable.

Beverly's brain contains, effectively, a broken warning device in its limbic system, an old fuse box in which the fuses tend to melt for no good reason, emphatically declaring an emergency where none now exists.

Surprisingly, she will probably not wonder about or even remember the intense perceptual and emotional "warnings," because by the next heartbeat, a long-entrenched dissociative reaction to the declared emergency may already have been tripped in her brain, to "protect" her from this "unbearable" childhood memory. She may feel strangely angry, or paranoid, or childishly timid. Or instead she may feel that she has begun to move in an uncomfortably hazy dream world, far away and derealized. Or she may completely depart from her "self" for a while, continue to act, but without self-awareness. Should this last occur in a minor way, her total experience may be something such as, "Today when I was going to work, the train pulled into the station—the blasted thing is so loud!—and the next thing I remember, it was stopping at my stop." She may even be mildly amused at herself for her spaciness.

Most of us do not notice these experiences very much. They are more or less invisible to us as we go about daily life, and so we do not understand how much of daily life is effectively spent in the past, in reaction to the darkest hours we have known, nor do we comprehend how swampy and vitality-sucking some of our memories really are. Deepening the mire of our divided awareness, in the course of a lifetime such "protective" mental reactions acquire tremendous *habit strength*. These over-exercised muscles can take us away even when traumatic memory fragments have not been evoked. Sometimes dissociation can occur when we are simply confused or frustrated or nervous, whether we recognize our absences or not.

Typically, only those with the most desperate trauma histories are ever driven to discover and perhaps modify their absences from the present. Only the addictions, major depressions, suicide attempts, and general ruination that attend the most severe trauma disorders can sometimes supply motivation sufficiently fierce to run the gauntlet thrown down by insight and permanent change. On account of our neurological wiring, confronting past traumas requires one to reendure all of their terrors mentally, in their original intensity, to feel as if the worst nightmare had come true and the horrors had returned. All the brain's authoritative warnings against staying present for the memories and the painful emotions, all the faulty fuses, have to be deliberately ignored, and in cases of extreme or chronic past trauma, this process is nothing short of heroic.

It helps to have an awfully good reason to try, such as suffocating depression or some other demonic psychological torment. Perhaps this is a part of the reason why philosophers and theologians through the centuries have observed such a strong connection between unbearable earthly sorrow and spiritual enlightenment, a timeless relationship that psychologists have mysteriously overlooked.

In order to appreciate what psychological trauma can do to the mind, and to a life, let us consider an extreme case of divided awareness, that of a woman whose psyche was mangled by profound trauma in her past, and who came to me for treatment after several serious suicide attempts. Her story is far grimmer than any most of us will ever know, and the consequent suffering in her adult life has been nearly unsurvivable. And yet, should one meet her on the street, or know her only casually, she would seem quite normal. In fact, one might easily view her as enviable. Certainly, when looking on from a distance, nothing at all would appear to be wrong, and much would be conspicuously right.

Julia is brilliant. After the *summa cum laude* from Stanford, and the full scholarship at the graduate school in New York, she became an award-winning producer of documentary films. I met her when she was thirty-two, and an intellectual force to be reckoned with. A conversation with her reminds me of the *New York Review of Books*, except that she is funnier, and also a living, breathing human being who wears amethyst jewelry to contrast with her electric auburn hair. Her ultramarine eyes gleam, even when she is depressed, giving one the impression, immediately upon meeting her, that there is something special about her. She is, however, soft-spoken and disarming in the extreme. She does not glorify, does not even seem to notice, either her prodigious intelligence or her beauty.

Those same blue eyes notice everything, instantly, photographically. The first time she walked into my office, she said, "Oh how nice. Did you get that little statue in Haiti? I did a kind of project there once. What a spellbinding place!"

She was referring to a small soapstone figurine, the rounded abstraction of a kneeling man, that I had indeed purchased in Port-au-Prince, and that sat on a shelf parallel to my office door. She had not glanced back in that direction as she came in, and must have captured and processed the image in a microsecond of peripheral perception.

"That's very observant," I said, whereupon she directed at me a smile so sparkling and so warm that, for just the barest moment, her lifelong depression cracked and vanished from the air around her, as if it had been nothing but a bubble. The radiance of her momentary smile caused me to blink, and I knew exactly then, even before the first session began, that if she would let me, I would do everything I could to keep this particular light from going out.

At a moment's notice, Julia can speak entertainingly and at length about film, music, multicultural psychology, African politics, theories of literary criticism, and any number of other subjects. Her memory for detail is beyond exceptional, and she has the storyteller's gift. When she is recounting information, or a story, her own intellectual fascination with it gives her voice the poised and expertly modulated quality of the narrator of a high-budget documentary about some especially wondrous endangered animals, perhaps Tibetan snow leopards. She speaks a few astutely inflected sentences, and then pauses, almost as if she is listening—and expects you to be listening—for the stealthy *crunch-crunch* of paws on the snow's crust.

Curious about this, I once asked her whether she were an actress as well as a filmmaker. She laughed, and replied that she could do first-rate narrative voice-overs, if she did say so herself, but had not a smidgen of real theatrical ability. In fact, she said, sometimes the people she worked with teased her good-naturedly about this minor chink in her armor.

At my first session with her, when I asked her why she had come to therapy, she spent thirty minutes telling me in cinematic detail about her recent attempt to kill herself, by driving to an isolated Massachusetts beach at three a.m. on a Tuesday in late January, and lying down by the surf. By so doing, she sincerely expected not to be found until well after she had frozen to death. Taking her omniscient narrator tone, intellectually intrigued by the memory, she described the circumstances of her unlikely accidental rescue by a group of drunken college students, and then spent the second thirty minutes of our hour together likening this near-death experience to the strangely impersonal distance from story one can achieve on film with certain authorial camera moves.

"By then, I was floating above myself, looking down, sort of waiting. And I know I couldn't actually have seen those kids, but I *felt* that I did. Over the sound of the waves, I don't think you can really *hear* footsteps in the sand, but still . . ."

And I strained to hear the *crunch-crunch*.

Therapy is a frightening thing, and people do not often seek it out because they are only mildly unhappy. In my work, and because of the high-risk individuals who are referred to me, it is not unusual for me to hear stories of attempted suicide from people I have only just met. I have come almost to expect such accounts, in fact.

At our second session, and in exactly the same tone she had used to describe her suicide attempt, Julia began by giving me an interesting account of her new project on the life of a promising writer who had died young, reportedly of a rare blood disease he had contracted in western China. After about fifteen minutes of this, I stopped her, and explained that I wanted to know something about her, about Julia herself, rather than about Julia's work. Seeing the blank expression come over her face, I tried to provide her with some nonthreatening guidance. I asked her some general, factual questions about her childhood.

And at that second session, this is what the articulate, intellectually gifted Julia remembered about her own childhood: An only child, she knew that she had been born in Los Angeles, but she did not know in which hospital. She vaguely remembered that when she was about ten, her parents had moved with her to another neighborhood; but she did not remember anything about the first neighborhood, or even where it was. Though she did not know for sure, she assumed that the move must have taken place because her parents had become more prosperous. She remembered that she had a friend in high school named Barbara (with whom "I must have spent a lot of time"), but she could not remember Barbara's last name, or where Barbara had gone after high school. I asked Julia about her teachers, and she could not remember a single one of them, not from grade school, not from middle school, not from high school. She could not remember whether or not she had gone to her high school prom or her high school graduation. The only thing she seemed to remember vividly from childhood was that when she was about twelve, she had a little terrier dog named Grin, and that her mother had Grin put to sleep when he needed an expensive stomach operation.

And that was all she remembered of her childhood, this successful thirty-two-year-old woman with the cinematic mind. And it took forty-five minutes for her to pull out that much from the dark, silent place that housed her early memories. She could not remember a single holiday or a single birthday. At thirty-two, she could swim, read, drive a car, and play a few songs on the piano. But she could not remember learning any of these skills.

Insufficient memory in the context of an adequate intellect, let alone a gifted one, is the next observation—right after the extraordinary understatement and humor—that causes me to become suspicious about a patient's past.

At our third session, she asked me an astonishing question, but also, really, the obvious question: "Do other people remember those things, about their teachers, and going to their graduation, and learning to drive, and so on?" When I told her that, yes, they usually do remember, at least to a much greater degree than she did, she reverently said, "Wow," and then she was quiet for a few minutes. Finally, she leaned forward a little and asked, "So what's wrong with me?"

Cautiously, because I knew what I had to say might at first sound preposterous or worse to Julia, I said, "I'm wondering about early traumatic experiences in your life. Even when someone's cognitive memory is perfectly good, as yours is, trauma can disrupt the memory in emotional ways."

Julia thought I was way off base; or at least the part of her that collected amethyst jewelry, made award-winning films, and talked about camera angles thought I was way off base. Another part of Julia, the part that kept trying to commit suicide, the part that prevented her from moving back to Los Angeles as her career demanded, the part that sometimes made her so sleepy during the middle of an ordinary day that she had to be driven home, that part kept her coming back to therapy for the next six years. During those six years, step by step, Julia and I cast some light on what had happened to her. She agreed to be hypnotized; she began to remember her dreams; she acknowledged her faint suspicions. She even traveled back to Los Angeles, to talk with distant relatives and old neighbors.

What we eventually discovered was that, when she was a child, Julia had lived in a house of horrors, with monsters jumping out at her without warning and for no apparent reason, except that Julia had come to assume, as abused children do, that she must be a horrible person who deserved these punishments. By the time she was school age, she had learned not to cry, because tears only encouraged her parents to abuse her further. Also, she had lost any inclination whatsoever to let anyone know what was going on. Telling someone and asking for help were concepts foreign to her despairing little soul. The thought that her life might be different had simply stopped occurring to her.

And soon, in a sense, she had stopped telling even herself. When the abuse began, she would "go somewhere else"; she would "not be there." By this, she meant that her mind had learned how to dissociate Julia's self from what was going on around her, how to transport her awareness to a place far enough away that, at most, she felt she was watching the life of a little girl named Julia from a very great distance. A sad little girl named Julia was helpless and could not escape; but psychologically, Julia's self could go "somewhere else," could be psychologically absent.

Simply put, Julia did not remember her childhood because she was not present for it.

All human beings have the capacity to dissociate psychologically, though most of us are unaware of this, and consider "out of body" episodes to be far beyond the boundaries of our normal experience. In fact, dissociative experiences happen to everyone, and most of these events are quite ordinary.

Consider a perfectly ordinary person as he walks into a perfectly ordinary movie theater to see a popular movie. He is awake, alert, and oriented to his surroundings. He is aware that his wife is with him and that, as they sit down in their aisle seats, she is to his right. He is aware that he has a box of popcorn on his lap. He knows that the movie he has come to see is entitled *The Fugitive*, and that its star is Harrison Ford, an actor. As he waits for the movie to begin, perhaps he worries about a problem he is having at work.

Then the lights in the theater are lowered, and the movie starts. And within twenty-five minutes, he has utterly lost his grasp on reality. Not only is he no longer worried about work, he no longer realizes that he has a job. If one could read his thoughts, one would discover that he no longer believes he is sitting in a theater, though in reality, he is. He cannot smell his popcorn; some of it tumbles out of the box he now holds slightly askew, because he has forgotten about his own hands. His wife has vanished, though any observer would see that she is still seated four inches to his right.

And without moving from his own seat, he is running, running, running—not with Harrison Ford, the actor—but with the beleaguered fugitive in the movie, with, in other words, a person who does not exist at all, in this moviegoer's real world or anyone else's. His heart races as he dodges a runaway train that does not exist, either.

This perfectly ordinary man is dissociated from reality. Effectively, he is in a trance. We might label his perceptions as psychotic, except for the fact that when the movie is over, he will return to his usual mental status almost instantly. He will see the credits. He will notice that he has spilled some popcorn, although he will not remember doing so. He will look to his right and speak to his wife. More than likely, he will tell her that he liked the movie, as we all tend to enjoy entertainments in which we can become lost. All that really happened is that, for a little while, he took the part of himself that worries about work problems and other "real" things, and separated it from the imaginative part of himself, so that the imaginative part could have dominance. He *dissociated* one part of his consciousness from another part.

When dissociation is illustrated in this way, most people can acknowledge that they have had such interludes from time to time, at a movie or a play, reading a book or hearing a speech, or even just daydreaming. And then the out-of-body may sound a little closer to home. Plainly stated, it is the case that under certain circumstances, ranging from pleasant or unpleasant distraction to fascination to fear to pain to horror, a human being can be psychologically absent from his or her own direct experience. We can go somewhere else. The part of consciousness that we nearly always conceive of as the "self" can be not there for a few moments, for a few hours, and in heinous circumstances, for much longer.

As the result of a daydream, this mental compartmentalization is called distraction. As the result of an involving movie, it is often called escape. As the result of trauma, physical or psychological, it is called a dissociative state. When a hypnotist induces dissociation, by monotony, distraction, relaxation or any number of other methods, the temporary result is called an hypnotic state, or a trance. The physiological patterns and the primary behavioral results of distraction, escape, dissociative state, and trance are virtually identical, regardless of method. The differences among them seem to result not so much from how consciousness gets divided as from how often and how long one is forced to keep it divided.

Another recognizable example of how consciousness can be split into pieces has to do with the perception of physical pain. On the morning after seeing *The Fugitive*, our moviegoer's wife is working frenetically to pack her briefcase, eat her breakfast, get the kids off to school, and listen to a news report on television, all at the same time. She is very distracted. In the process of all this, she bashes her leg soundly against the corner of a low shelf. Yet the woman is not seemingly aware that she has injured herself. That night, as she is getting ready for bed, she notices that she has a large colorful bruise on her right thigh. She thinks, "Well, now, I wonder how I did that."

In this case, a person was distracted, and the part of her consciousness that would normally have perceived pain was split apart from, and subjugated to, the part of her consciousness that was goal-directed. She was not there for the direct experience of her pain. She was somewhere else (the briefcase, the breakfast, the kids, the news). And because she was not there, she does not remember the accident.

The direct experience of physical pain can be split off in cases of much more serious injury as well. Most of us have heard stories along the lines of the parent who, with a broken leg, goes back to the scene of an accident and wrenches open a mangled car door with her bare hands in order to rescue her child. Less valorous, I myself remember my car being demolished by a speeding limousine. My knee was injured, but I felt no pain just after the crash, was more or less unaware of my body at all. My first thought before being dragged out of my car was to peer into the rearview mirror and inspect my teeth, and to decide that everything must be okay because there were no chips in them. And then there are the war stories about maimed infantrymen who have had to flee from the front line. All such circumstances affect memory in fascinating ways. Note, for example, that when veterans get together, they often laugh and tell war stories as though those times had been the best of their lives.

Agony that is psychological can be dissociated, too. While she was being abused, Julia developed the reaction of standing apart from herself and her situation. She stopped being there. Certainly, some parts of her consciousness must have been there right along. She could watch her parents, even predict their moods. She could run and hide. She could cover her injuries. She could keep her parents' secrets. But the part of her consciousness that she thinks of as her self was not there; it was split off, put aside, and therefore in some sense protected. And because her self had not been there, her self could not remember what had happened to her during much of her childhood.

What does this feel like, not being able to remember whole chapters of one's own life? I have asked many people this question, Julia among them. As usual, her answer was obvious and startling at the same time.

"It doesn't feel like anything," she answered. "I never really thought about it. I guess I just assumed, sort of tacitly assumed, that everyone's memory was like mine, that is to say, kind of blank before the age of twenty or so. I mean, you can't see into someone else's mind, right? All you can do is ask questions, and it never even occurred to me to ask anybody about this. It's like asking, 'What do you see when you see blue?' First of all, you'd never think to ask. And secondly, two people can agree that the clear blue sky is blue, but does the actual color blue look the *same* to both of them? Who knows? How would you even ask that question?

"Of course, every now and then I'd hear people talking about pin-the-tail-on-the-donkey, or some other thing about a little kid's birthday, and I'd wonder how they knew that. But I guess I just figured their memory was especially good, or maybe they'd heard their parents talk about it so much that it seemed like a memory.

"The memories I did have seemed like aberrations, like pin-points of light in a dark room, so vague that you're not really sure whether you're seeing them or not. Certainly, there was nothing like a continuous thread of memory that linked one part of my life to another.

"Really it wasn't until you started asking me questions about my teachers and so forth that I ever even had any serious questions about my memory. After you started asking, I asked a couple of other people, just out of curiosity, and I began to realize that other people really do have childhood memories, and some of them are pretty vivid. I was surprised.

"What can I tell you? It just never occurred to me to wonder about it before. It felt like . . . it felt like nothing."

She shrugged. Most people shrug. They are genuinely surprised, and at a loss.

Now the conspicuous question to ask Julia was, "All this time that you've been so unhappy, all the times you've tried to end your life, what did you think was causing all that misery?"

"I thought I was crazy," she answered.

This is easy enough to understand. Imagine a simple and, relatively speaking, innocuous example. Imagine that someone, call her Alice, leaves work early one day and goes to the oral surgeon to have her two bottom wisdom teeth extracted. The extractions go well; the doctor packs the gums with cotton and sends Alice home. On the way home, for some fictitious reason, let us say magic moonbeams, Alice completely loses her memory of the visit to the oral surgeon. She now assumes that she is driving directly home from work, as she does on most days. After she gets home, she is okay for a while, but gradually the anesthetic wears off, and she begins to experience a considerable amount of pain in her mouth. Soon the pain is too strong to ignore, and she goes to the bathroom mirror to examine the situation. When she looks into her mouth, she discovers that there are wads of cotton in there. And when she takes the cotton out, she discovers that two of her teeth are missing, and she is bleeding!

Alice is now in the twilight zone. The ordinary experience of having her wisdom teeth pulled has turned into a situation that makes her feel insane. One or two more of such experiences, and she would be convinced.

Childhood trauma creates a particularly bewildering picture.

Observe normal children at play, and you will realize that children are especially good at dissociating. In the interest of play, a child can, in a heartbeat, leave himself behind, become someone or something else, or several things at once. Reality is even more plastic in childhood. Pretend games are real and wonderful and consuming. It is clear to anyone who really looks that normal children derive unending joy from their superior ability to leap out of their "selves" and go somewhere else, be other things. The snow is not cold. The body is not tired, even when it is on the verge of collapse.

Because children dissociate readily even in ordinary circumstances, when they encounter traumatic situations, they easily split their consciousness into pieces, often for extended periods of time. The self is put aside and hidden. Of course, this reaction is functional for the traumatized child, necessary, even kind. For the traumatized child, a dissociative state, far from being dysfunctional or crazy, may in fact be lifesaving. And thanks be to the normal human mind that it provides the means.

This coping strategy becomes dysfunctional only later, after the child is grown and away from the original trauma. When the original trauma is no longer an ongoing fact of life, prolonged dissociative reactions are no longer necessary. But through the years of intensive use, the self-protective strategy has developed a hair trigger. The adult whom the child has become now experiences dissociative reactions to levels of stress that probably would not cause another person to dissociate.

The events that are most problematic tend to be related in some way to the original trauma. However, human beings are exquisitely symbolic creatures, and "related" can reach unpredictable and often indecipherable levels of abstraction and metaphor. A long shadow from a city streetlight can remind someone of the tall cacti on the Arizona desert where his father used to threaten to "feed" him to the rattlesnakes. An innocent song about the wind in the willow trees can remind someone else of the rice fields that were a part of her childhood's landscape in Cambodia. A car backfiring on

Beacon Street in Boston can remind yet another person of that spot on the trail where his eighteen-year-old platoon mate exploded six feet in front of him.

And so for the adult who was traumatized as a child, the present too has a kind of mercurial quality. The present is difficult to hold on to, always getting away.

In Julia's case, though she had not questioned her poverty of memory for the past, she had begun to suspect even before she came into therapy that she was losing time in the present. Probably this is because there are more external reality checks on the present than there are on the past. From other people—and from radio, television, the Internet, date books—there are ongoing reminders of the present time of day, and day of the week. Markers of time in the past are less immediate, and sooner or later most dates and chronologies for the past begin to feel amorphous to us all. It is hardly amazing that one should have forgotten something that happened twenty years ago. But if a person lets on that she has no memory of an important event that occurred this very week, friends and associates are unlikely to let such a lapse go unremarked.

At one of her early sessions with me, Julia announced, "When I woke up Tuesday morning it was Friday."

"Pardon?"

"When I woke up this morning it was Tuesday, and then I discovered that it was Friday for everybody else."

"How do you mean?"

"Well, the last thing I remember before waking up this morning was having dinner Monday night. So I thought it was Tuesday. And then I went in to work, and some sponsors were there that I was supposed to meet with on Friday. So I asked my assistant what was up, and she said, 'You wanted to meet with these people this morning, remember?' And I said, 'No. I wanted to meet with them on Friday.' She looked at me, and said, 'Today is Friday, Julia.'

"I finessed. I laughed and said, 'Of course. That's terrible. No more late nights for me. Pretty soon I'll be forgetting my name.

Ha, ha.' But it isn't funny. This happens a lot. I just lose time. Hours, days. They're gone, and I don't know what I've done or where I've been or anything else.

"I've never told anyone this before. It's embarrassing. Actually, it's terrifying.

"I don't understand any of it, but the thing I understand the least is that apparently I go about my business during these times, and nobody notices any difference in me. At least, no one ever says anything. After the meeting this morning, I realized that on Tuesday, Wednesday, and Thursday, I must have done a mountain of editing. There it was, all finished. I did a good job, even. And I don't remember a bloody thing."

During this confession, I saw Julia cry for the first time. Quickly, though, she willed her tears under control, and wanted me to tell her about a word she had heard me use the previous week, "dissociative." She questioned me as if the issue were a strictly academic one for her, which it clearly was not. I gently steered her back to the subject of herself and her week.

"Where did you have dinner Monday night?"

"What? Oh. Dinner Monday night. I had dinner at the Grill 23 with my friend Elaine."

"Was it a nice time?" I continued to question.

"I think so. Yes, I think it was okay."

"What did you and Elaine talk about, do you remember?"

"What did we talk about? Let's see. Well, I think we talked about the film a bit. And we talked about the waiter. Very cute waiter." She grinned. "And we probably spent the longest time talking about Elaine's relationship with this new guy, Peter. Why do you ask?"

"You said the dinner was the last thing you remembered before you woke up this morning. I thought it might be important. What did Elaine say about Peter?"

"Well, she said she's madly in love, and she said she wanted me to meet him because she thought we'd have a lot to talk about. He's from L.A., too."

"You and Peter are both from L.A. What else did you and Elaine say about L.A.?"

Julia looked suddenly blank, and said, "I don't remember. Why? Do you really think something about the place where I grew up scares me enough that just talking about it blasts me into never-never land for three days? That really can't be, though. I mean, I talk about L.A. a lot to people."

"I think it's possible that something during the dinner scared you enough to make you lose yourself for a while, although we'll never know for sure. Obviously, talking about L.A. doesn't always do that, but maybe there was something in that particular conversation that reminded you of something else that triggered something in your mind, something that might seem innocuous to another person, or even to you at another time. But as I say, we'll never know for sure."

"That's frightening. That's awful. It's like I'm in jail in my own head. I don't think I can live this way anymore."

"Yes, it's very frightening. I suspect it's been very frightening for a long time."

"You got that right."

Julia's knowledge of her own life, both past and present, had assumed the airy structure of Swiss cheese, with some solid substance that she and her gifted intellect could use, but riddled with unexplained gaps and hollows. This had its funny side. A few months later, when she had gained a better acceptance of her problem, she came in, sat down, and said in a characteristically charming way, "How do you like my new bracelet?"

"It's beautiful," I replied. "I've always admired your amethyst jewelry. When did you get that piece?"

"Who knows?"

She grinned at me again, and we both laughed.

The somewhat old-fashioned term for Julia's departures from herself during which she would continue to carry out day-to-day activities is "fugue," from the Italian word *fuga*, meaning "flight." A dissociative state that reaches the point of fugue is one of the most dramatic spontaneously occurring examples of the human mind's ability to divide consciousness into parts. In fugue, the person, or the mind of the person, can be subdivided in a manner that allows certain intellectually driven functions to continue—rising at a certain time, conversing with others, following a schedule, even carrying out complex tasks—while the part of consciousness that we usually experience as the "self"—the self-aware center that wishes, dreams, plans, emotes, and remembers—has taken flight, or has perhaps just darkened like a room at night when someone is sleeping.

The departures of fugue are related to certain experiences in ordinary human life that are not generated by trauma. For example, similar is the common experience of the daily commuter by car who realizes that sometimes she or he arrives back at home in the evening without having been aware of the activities of driving. The driving was automatically carried out by some part of the mind, while the self part of the mind was worrying, daydreaming, or listening to the radio. The experience is that of arriving at home without remembering the process of the trip. If one reflects upon the minute and complex decisions and maneuvers involved in driving a car, this ordinary event is really quite remarkable.

Clinical fugue differs from common human experience not so much in kind as in degree. Fugue is terror-driven and complete, while the more recognizable condition is the result of distraction, and relatively transparent. As fugue, the car trip example would involve a driver who failed to remember not just the process of the trip, but also the fact that there had been a trip, and from where. Far beyond distraction, the more remarkable dissociative reaction of fugue would have been set off by something—an event, a conversation, an image, a thought—that was related, though perhaps in some oblique and symbolic way, to trauma.

Not all traumatized individuals exhibit outright fugue. For some people, stressful events trigger a demifugue that is less dramatic but in some ways more agonizing. Another of my patients, Lila, refers to her experience as "my flyaway self":

"I had an argument with the cashier at the Seven-Eleven store. I gave him a twenty and he said I gave him a ten. He wouldn't give me my other ten dollars back. The way he looked at me—it was just the way my stepfather used to, like I was stupid, like I was dirt. I knew he wasn't really my stepfather, but all the feelings were there anyway. After a minute, I just couldn't argue about it. I left without my money, and by the time I got back home, my flyaway self thing had started. Once it starts, it's like there's absolutely nothing I can do about it. I'm gone, and there's nothing I can do about it."

"What does it feel like?"

"Oh boy. I don't know how to describe it. It's just . . . it's just really awful. I don't know . . . everything around me gets very small, kind of unreal, you know? It's my flyaway self, I call it. It feels like . . . my spirit just kind of flies away, and everything else gets very small—people, everything. If it were happening now, for example, you would look very small and far away, and the room would feel kind of unreal. Sometimes even my own body gets small and unreal. It's awful. And when it happens, I can't stop it. I just can't stop it."

What Lila describes as her "flyaway self" is in some respects similar to the derealization that most people have known occasionally, usually under passing conditions of sleep deprivation or physical illness. One temporarily has the sense of looking at the world through the wrong end of a telescope: everything looks small and far away, though one knows intellectually that these same things are just as close and life-sized as ever.

Imagine being forced to live lengthy segments of your life in this state. Imagine that you were falling inexorably into it, to remain there for a week or more at a time, because of events such as an unpleasant argument with a stranger at a convenience store. As bad as this would be, the situation for someone like Lila is incalculably worse, because for her the phenomenon has its origins in trauma.

Another of my patients offered a specific image, and for me an indelible one, to describe the same dissociative condition. Forty-nine-year-old Seth, like Julia, is successful, educated, and visually talented, and his disquieting description reflects his aptitudes. At the beginning of this particular therapy session, he had been telling me about a startling encounter, at a company softball game, with another person lost in the dissociated space with which he himself was all too familiar.

"I knew exactly where she was," said Seth.

"What does it feel like?" I asked. "Can you tell me what it feels like when you're there? How do you change?"

"I don't change. It's not that I change. *Reality* changes. Everything becomes very small, and I exist entirely inside my mind. Even my own body isn't real."

Indicating the two of us and the room around us, he continued, "Right now, this is what's real. You're real. What we're saying is real. But when I'm like that, the office is not real. *You're* not real anymore."

"What is real at those times?" I asked.

"I don't know exactly. It's hard to explain. Only what's going on in my mind is real. I'll tell you what it feels like: I feel like I'm dog-paddling out in the ocean, moving backwards, out to sea. When I'm still close enough to the land, I can sort of look way far away and see the beach. You and the rest of the world are all on the beach somewhere. But I keep drifting backwards, and the beach gets smaller, and the ocean gets bigger and bigger, and when I've drifted out far enough, the beach disappears, and all I can see all around me is the sea. It's so gray—gray on gray on gray."

"Is there anything out in the ocean with you?" I asked.

Seth replied, "No. Not at that point. I'm completely alone, more alone than you can imagine. But if you drift out farther, if you go all the way out to where the bottom of the sea drops off to the real abyss part, then there are awful things, these bloodthirsty sea creatures, sharks and giant eels and things like that. I've always thought that if something in the real world scared me enough, I'd drift out and out to past the dropping-off part, and then I would just be gobbled up, gone—no coming back, ever.

"When I'm floating out in the middle of the sea, everything else is very far away, even time. Time becomes unreal, in a way. An hour could go by that seems like a day to me, or four or five hours could go by, and it seems like only a minute."

Some extreme trauma survivors recognize that they are dissociative, and others do not recognize this. Many times, an individual will realize at some point in adulthood that she or he has had a lifelong pattern of being "away" a grievously large portion of the time.

During the same session, Seth described his own situation in this way:

"Actually, when I was a child, I don't know how much time I spent away like that. I never thought about it. It was probably a lot of the time, maybe even all the time. It just *was*."

"You mean it was your reality, and so of course you never questioned it, any more than any other child questions his reality?"

"Right. That's right. That was when I was a child. And most of the time it still happens automatically, bang, way before I know it's coming; but in here now, sometimes, there's this brief moment when I know I'm about to go away, but I still have time to try to keep it from taking over. Emphasis on *try*."

"How do you do that?" I asked.

"By concentrating. By trying with everything I've got to concentrate on you, and what you're saying, and on the things around me in the office here. But then there's physical pain, too. My eyes hurt, and I know I could make myself feel better if I shut them. But I try not to. And I get this thing in my stomach, which is the hardest thing to fight. There's this pain that feels like I just swallowed a whole pile of burning coals, this torture feeling that beams out from my stomach to the rest of my body; sooner or later, it just takes me over."

He grimaced and put a fist to his breastbone.

When Seth said this about pain in his stomach, I remembered, as I had remembered during descriptions by many, many others, that there is a common Japanese term, *shin pan*, inexactly translated as "agitated heart syndrome," referring to a great pain between the chest and the stomach, just under the solar plexus. *Shin pan*, a condition as real within Eastern medicine as is cataract or ulcer or fractured fibula within Western medicine, is a pain of the heart that does not involve the actual physical organ. In our culture, we consider such a thing—a "heartache," if you will—to be poetry at most. We do not understand that much of the rest of the world considers it to be quite real.

I said to Seth, "It must be frightening to be out in the ocean like that."

"Actually, it's not," he replied. "The abyss part, with the sharks and all, that's frightening. But for most of my life it was really no more frightening than the things that were on the beach, no more frightening than reality, I guess is what I'm saying. So floating in the middle of the ocean was really the best place, even though I guess that sounds strange. Also, being there takes care of the physical pain; there's no more pain when I'm there. It's just that now, I mean lately, the beach, where you are, and everything else, sometimes it makes me wish I could maybe be there instead. I guess you could say that now, at least sometimes, I want to live."

I smiled at him, but he looked away, unsure of what he had just proposed.

Referring back to Seth's softball team acquaintance, whose dissociative episode had begun our discussion, I said, "It must be strange to be with another person when you know she's drifting away in an ocean just like you do sometimes."

"Yes, it's very strange."

"How did you know she was drifting? Did she tell you?"

"No. She didn't tell me. She didn't say anything at all about being dissociated. She was just standing around with us, talking about these incredible things, horrible things from her past, without any emotion, without any reaction to them. She played well that day, actually, but she won't remember any of it, that's for sure."

"You mean," I asked, "another person, besides you, might not have known she was dissociated?"

"Absolutely. I'm sure someone else might not have known at all. It's just that I looked at her, and I saw me. It was like talking to somebody who didn't have a soul."

"You mean her soul was somewhere else?"

"Yes, I guess so. Her soul was somewhere else," Seth said.

After a brief silence, he turned the discussion back to his own life: "The other day, my wife was trying to talk to me about something really important that happened when the twins were born. Doesn't matter what it was; what matters is that I had no idea what she was talking about. I didn't have a clue. It wasn't a dim memory. It wasn't anything. I didn't have that memory because I wasn't there."

"You weren't there, but your wife didn't know that at the time?" I asked.

"No, she didn't know that at all. But you know, most of the time when she and I are making love, and I'm not there, she doesn't know it even then."

"You mean, someone can be that close to you, and still not know?"

"Yes."

At that moment I thought, and then decided to say aloud, "That's so sad."

A single tear skimmed down Seth's cheek. He wiped it quickly with the back of his hand, and said, "I'm sorry, it's just that, well, when I think about it, I realize that, really, I've missed most of my own life."

He stopped and took a deep breath, and I wondered whether he might have to dissociate just to get through this experience in my office.

I asked, "Are you here now, at this moment?"

"Yes, I think so. Yes."

There was another pause, and then with more emotion in his

voice than he was usually able to show, he said, "It's so hard, because so much of the time when I'm here, what you're seeing is not
what I'm seeing. I feel like such an impostor. I'm out in my ocean,
and you don't know that. And I can't tell you what's going on.
Sometimes I'd really like to tell you, but I can't. I'm gone."

Seth's description of his inner life makes it wrenchingly clear that
the traumatized person is unable to feel completely connected to
another person, even a friend, even a spouse. Just as limiting, perhaps even more limiting, is such a person's disconnection from his
or her own body. You will recall that Lila's "flyaway self" owned a
body that was only "small and unreal," and that when Seth was in
his ocean, his mind was separated from his physical self. I began
this chapter with Julia, the brilliant producer of documentary
films, and as it happens, about a year into her treatment, an event
occurred that well illustrates the survivor's trauma-generated dissociation from the body itself, or more accurately, from those aspects of mind that inform one of what is going on in the body.

One morning just after the workday began, Julia's assistant, a
gentle young woman who was quite fond of her boss, noticed that
Julia was looking extremely pale. She asked how Julia was feeling,
and Julia replied that she thought her stomach was a little upset,
but other than that she was sure she was fine. Ten minutes later,
walking down a corridor, Julia fell to the floor, and by the time the
panic-stricken assistant came to her aid, she was unconscious. An
ambulance arrived and rushed Julia to the Massachusetts General
Hospital, where she underwent an immediate emergency appen-
dectomy. Her life was in danger, and the situation was touch-and-
go for a while, because her infected appendix had already ruptured
and severe peritonitis had resulted. She survived, however, and
during her recovery, when she was well enough to see me again,
she recounted a postsurgery conversation with her doctor.

"The doctor kept asking me, 'Didn't you feel anything? Weren't you in pain?' I told her my stomach had been upset that morning, but I didn't remember any real pain. She said, 'Why didn't you call me?' I guess she just couldn't believe that I really hadn't felt any pain. She said that I should have been in agony by the previous night, at the very latest. She kept saying 'agony.' But I didn't feel it. I swear to you I didn't feel any pain, much less agony."

"I believe you," I said to Julia.

"Well, I don't think she did. I guess a ruptured appendix involves a lot of pain for most people."

"Yes. Yes it does," I replied, trying to disguise some of my own astonishment.

"I know I've tried to kill myself intentionally, more than once, so maybe this sounds crazy—but I don't want to die one day just because I'm confused."

"What do you mean?" I asked.

"I don't want to die because I can't feel anything. I don't want to end up dead because I can't feel what's going on in my body, or because I can't tell the difference between that psychosomatic pain I'm always getting in my chest and some honest-to-God heart attack."

Julia said "psychosomatic," but I was thinking *shin pan*, again.

"You know how we talk about my tendency to be dissociative? Well do you think I dissociate from my body too? Because if that's what I'm doing, then it's the illusion from hell. I mean, if it's supposed to save me, it's not working. In fact, it's going to kill me one day. And even if it doesn't kill me, what's the use of living if I can't feel anything? Why should I be alive when I lose big parts of my life? I mean, really, how can you care about anything if you can't even know the truth about yourself? If you keep losing yourself?"

I said, "I think that's one of the best questions I've ever heard."

"You do? You mean you agree with me about how I can't really care about living if I keep losing myself?"

"I said that's one of the best *questions*. I didn't say I knew the answer."

"Oh boy, you're cagey," she said, and grinned. "So okay, how do I find the answer?"

"Well you know, you could try to remember. We could try hypnosis, for one thing."

I believed that Julia might be ready to bring up the lights in the cold, dark house of her past.

"Yes, so you've said. And the idea scares the hell out of me." There was a substantial pause before she continued. "The idea scares the hell out of me, but I think I have to do it anyway."

"Why do you have to?"

"Because I want to know. Because I want to live."

"So, let's do it?" I asked.

"Let's do it," Julia said.

PART TWO

THE SHELL-SHOCKED SPECIES

CHAPTER THREE

Duck and Cover

Probably no adult misery can be compared with a child's despair.

—Iris Murdoch

When he was living in California, my brother, Steve, my wise mentor in so many things, offered to escort his visiting sister to Año Nuevo State Reserve, a destination not far south of San Francisco, between Santa Cruz and Half Moon Bay. We drove the fifty-five miles in no time, and then hiked three more miles to see the colony of northern elephant seals, magnificent rare beasts that the state of California is trying to save from extinction. The hike took us across an eerie, otherworldy terrain—a windy, barren expanse of sand dunes—even more alien for being so close to the crowds of San Francisco.

The party we joined included a park ranger, six other adults, and, with two of these, a bright-eyed, towheaded four-year-old boy. We were all curious about the elephant seals, but none of us was so excited as the child, who kept asking the ranger whether or not we would be able to pet the seals. The ranger explained to him several times that we would be able to look at the seals, but we could not touch them.

When we reached the stark Pacific beach, the seals were there in force. An adult elephant seal is a furry, limbless being that weighs approximately two tons. It looks like a car-sized protozoan that has for some reason been wrapped in a stringy brown-gray carpet. The carpet appears to be pitifully afflicted with mange. Great hunks of it are peeling off, or missing altogether. And an elephant seal stinks, in about the way one would expect a limbless and immobilized two-ton molting mammal to stink. A large group of elephant seals smells something like a newly fertilized field.

We heard the seals before we saw them. They roared like angry jungle cats, and when they saw us, their roars became more furious. The ranger had already explained that, unfortunately, elephant seals do not like human beings very much. However, these enormous formless creatures cannot give chase on land—except for the tedious inches at a time they gain by rocking from side to side like hammock-sized bags of pudding—and therefore we could approach within ten feet or so. While we stood back and stared, the whiskered seal faces on the gigantic pudding bodies reflected the rage of impotence.

But the little boy's face was transformed with joy, and all the good intentions of friendship. He pulled on the park ranger's arm.

"Do you hear those seals?" he asked conspiratorially, as if there could be some doubt.

"Yes I do," replied the ranger. "They make a lot of noise, don't they?"

Screwing up his face with an adult seriousness, the boy continued. "Do you know what they're saying?"

"Why no. What are they saying?"

"They're saying they want me to pet them. I can't stay back here anymore. The seals have got to be petted, okay?"

The poor man tried once again to explain the untenable fact that while we could look, we simply could not touch.

Later, Steve and I agreed that the child had been just as interesting as the exotic animals. He wept on the way back, because he had not been allowed to pet the snarling two-ton seals, and stopped crying only when the ranger found a graceful little green snake under some scrub, and placed it on the boy's open palm. The reptile looped delicately around the child's pale fingers, and then dropped to the ground between his feet, a sweet curl of green between two tiny Reeboks.

He was nearly transfixed with enchantment. "Can I have it?" he asked.

His parents looked at each other regretfully, and explained that he could not. The father knelt beside him and said, "Sweetie, I'm sorry, but you see, this little baby snake has got to go home now."

Children understand about home. The boy's face clouded again, but he picked up the snake and carefully put it back under its homey bit of scrub.

"See you later," he chided it hopefully, and we all continued our walk back to civilization, bringing with us the child, who would have lingered.

Since then, I often think about this little boy with his unedited awareness—wanting to talk to the monsters, to pat their mildewed fur, to be friends. His parents were loving and respectful, and life for him was an endless, immediate moment, no avoidance, no self-protective departures, and as yet, no fear. At Año Nuevo that day, I felt it [I think we all felt it—the nostalgic wish that the child could remain just as he was, the wish that life would not put out its claws and change him. And the vague dread too, knowing that this was not possible.]I remember that as we slowly hiked back across the dunes, the nine of us, including the ranger, all clustered around the little boy, or carried him, just exactly like what we really were: a small group of migrating animals instinctively guarding its young.

We, along with all other forms of life, are about the survival of our kind. Our bodies, our brains, our emotions, and our behavior all reflect this simple fact. Under stupendous pressures from the physical world they lived in, across time without memory, our ancestors' ancestors, skinny, threatened hominids, were selected for their quick, clear mental proclivities for keeping themselves alive: the instinct to protect their offspring against all comers, the instinct to stay together in groups, a fear of strangers. And survival was a formidable challenge. When our species began, the average newborn human probably had a chance to survive not much greater than that of a hatchling loggerhead turtle racing across a gull-canopied beach to the sea; our primordial past is one of just such fantastic assailability. Our bodies and our brains were forged in a white-hot fire, and even as we enter a new millennium, we remain the product of these ancient beginnings.

Like baby loggerheads, we needed to focus keenly on the task of attaining safe haven. But unlike turtles, we had evolved as complex creatures, cognitively astute, mentally representational, aware of the possibility of injury, pain, and death. We comprehended the actual dangers, and many of the potential ones. We considered, we planned, we dreamed, we dreaded. For all the obvious reasons, our mighty brains were a large advantage when it came to surviving our planet's hazards; and for their somewhat less conspicuous effects, our complex brains were a disadvantage too. As an analogy, imagine that a hatchling turtle develops an awareness that a seagull might well, within moments, crush its tiny shell and gobble its flesh. What would happen should this abrupt sentience cause the new reptile to freeze up in terror along its path to the sea rather than continuing its oblivious scurry? It would be killed instantly, of course. Never would it have the chance to lay its own turtle eggs.

In this way, sentience is both a blessing and a curse, where survival is concerned. Even nonhuman animals, when they sense predators within striking range, narrow their perceptual field, and have been shown to experience a convenient bodily analgesia when under attack. Human beings have mitigated the curse of their more advanced awareness with a variety of sophisticated dissociative capacities that often allow us to function effectively in terrifying circumstances. For instance, we can take mental departures, as Julia did, and we can go on moving, though our own unendurable monsters be in flight all around us. Julia's childhood mind was not freakish; on the contrary, it was precisely normal, the breath-takingly adaptive product of eons.

Our mental resiliency in petrifying circumstances is normal. But how normal are the desperate circumstances themselves? As we begin a new century, how common, really, are the monsters that beset human beings? How many of them are there still, in a technological age? Here is the answer, although be warned that it is not a pleasing one:

Often, now, the faces on the monsters are different; but we live in a world that still assaults the consciousness of all its children. That we do not all usually think of ourselves as having been traumatized is in part a tribute to the human spirit.

Child abuse, as in Julia's case, is but a bare beginning, though according to the National Committee to Prevent Child Abuse, about forty-seven out of every one thousand American children are reported as victims of child maltreatment, to our various child protective services. In a conservative estimate, reported or not, 38 percent of all girls and 16 percent of all boys are sexually abused before the age of eighteen.

For children to witness violence is an established feature of our lives. In the United States alone, medical expenses from domestic violence total three to five billion dollars a year. Leaving the home for our urban streets—in an American Psychological Association study of first- and second-graders in Washington, D.C., 45 percent said they had witnessed muggings, 31 percent said they had witnessed shootings, and 39 percent said they had seen dead bodies.

But outnumbering even these statistics is the situation of perfectly ordinary children, children from families who are not violent, and who do not live in the inner city. Even the children who are not intentionally abused, even those who are not directly exposed to crime, witness parental rages and arguments at home, and media coverage of the most horrible events in the outside world. In plain fact, the list of consciousness-assailing events that are witnessed or endured by even the most protected children is extremely long: serious accidents, car crashes, the illnesses and deaths of loved ones, the fear or reality of peer ridicule, petrifying medical procedures, devastating custody battles, predictions of nuclear annihilation or environmental collapse, macabre lessons in how to get away from the "stranger" whom protective parents are constantly expecting.

Then one must reflect upon other, more fundamental situations, for example, the essential vulnerability of living in a human body at all—unavoidable physical pain, and, for some, loss of body function or body parts through disease, accident, or genetic glitch. Or as another example, the daily struggles of human families all over the globe who fear for their well-being, emotional and physical, on account of an immutable characteristic such as race or ethnicity.

We live inside fragile bodies in a dangerous world, especially when we are children, and should we stop to take an account of our experiences, we would discover that although only some of us have been abused, no one among us is completely unscathed, not even in our technological age. But I have been discussing psychological trauma specifically, not danger or hurt in general. What is the definition of psychological trauma? What kinds of situations and events are traumatizing, as opposed to simply painful or frightening?

One of the most widely accepted and helpful definitions is provided by Alexander McFarlane and Giovanni de Girolamo of, respectively, the University of Adelaide, Australia, and the Department of Mental Health, Bologna, Italy. Writing about the distribution and determinants of post-traumatic reactions in human populations, McFarlane and de Girolamo state that, more than just frightening or painful, traumatic situations are "events that violate our existing ways of making sense of our reactions, structuring our perceptions of other people's behavior, and creating a framework for interacting with the world at large. In part, this is determined by our ability to anticipate, protect, and know ourselves." In other words, it is possible for one person to survive a disastrous neighborhood fire and be distraught but not traumatized, because her particular views of the world and of other people are not violated, and because she feels able to cope; and it is equally possible for another person to be traumatized by a space heater fire, because it so confounds her ideas of what can happen to her, and because the fire brings her face-to-face with her own helplessness.

By definition, a traumatic event, whether it be objectively tragic or not, opens in the mind a corridor to the apprehension of our essential helplessness and the possibility of death. A traumatic stressor is overwhelming not because it is colossal—for it may not be so to observers—but because it has a certain meaning for the individual.

Imagine two skydivers. Skydiver A has been practicing her sport for many years. Skydiver B is jumping out of a plane for the first time. At the usual moment, Skydiver A pulls the release to open her parachute. The parachute does not open. She is bemused by this, because she is an experienced parachute-packer, and she thinks that her chute should have operated. She will have to recheck her work when she gets to the ground. But she knows that she has an emergency chute for just such mishaps. She waits for another thirty seconds, enjoying the free fall, and then activates her emergency parachute, which opens immediately.

Skydiver B, at the moment she has been taught to do so, tugs on the release to open *her* parachute. The parachute does not open. She cannot believe this is happening. She thinks she is about to die. She perceives herself plummeting helplessly through space, and begins to scream, although the air sluicing past her erases the sound. For about thirty seconds, as her life rushes before her eyes, she struggles to find her emergency chute. Finally, she activates the backup device, and it opens immediately.

For Skydiver A, another dive. For Skydiver B, a traumatic event, nightmares and intrusive memories to come, perhaps for years. For an onlooker, two more or less identical scenes. For the participants, two very different meanings.

Meaning is the important thing. It determines whether or not the mental corridor to helplessness and death will open up, or remain shut and disregarded by us, as that channel usually does. And the meaning we ascribe to a threatening event is determined in part by "our ability to anticipate, protect, and know ourselves," as McFarlane and de Girolamo have put it. The more we can anticipate what is likely to happen next, the more we feel that we can protect ourselves, the more we know ourselves in general, the more inoculated we are against being traumatized by the frightening or the painful.

There is one extremely large group of people who have almost no history of anticipating events, virtually no chance of protecting themselves, and only the most minimal self-knowledge. These are children, of course. Because of their lack of experience in our world, children are traumatized far more frequently than we are. Circumstances that provoke mild anxiety in adults may easily generate life-or-death terror in children, because the very young have not yet created for themselves a usable "framework for interacting with the world at large." This temporary deficit is one of the most poignant and dangerous connotations of the expression "childhood innocence."

When I was three years old, the picture of the wolf in the Little Golden Books version of *Bambi* evoked a careening terror in me. Now, after an inestimable number of encounters with pictures, stories, forests, sharp teeth, surprises, and my own fear, and even a few experiences with actual and not-so-scary gray wolves, the same image arouses in me no emotional reaction at all, apart from a little nostalgia. As adults, we are seldom able to appreciate the full measure of our early naïveté. A tiny person has literally everything to learn: I have ten fingers; water is wet; my toys fall down and not up. And what is this planet like anyway, this one that I have landed on?

A person with so many unanswered questions is tender, and receptive like a flower in the morning. She is also at our mercy, and at risk.

To make matters even more excruciating for the young, the im-

mature cognitive capacities of early childhood make it difficult, often impossible, to create an articulate narrative from a threatening
event, after the fact. A young child cannot reflect upon and make
sense of a traumatic episode, let alone report it coherently to
someone who might help him attach words and meaning to what
occurred. Even the unfortunate novice skydiver could understand
what had happened to her, put a story together in her mind, and
have the relief of telling others, perhaps obsessively for a while,
about the most frightening thirty seconds of her life. There is no
such relief for a small child, who will likely suffer the aftermath of
a trauma in helpless silence, and remember his experience in emotions and bodily reactions, rather than in words.

So the alarming truth is that even good, caring, protective parents can be clueless regarding certain experiences suffered by their
children. Also, adults tend to minimize a child's terror, even when
they are aware of its cause, simply because the source may seem innocuous to people with greater worldliness. For a child, it is overwhelming to see a drooling wolf menace Bambi; for an adult, it is
just another page in a children's storybook.

Focusing on children who are not abuse victims (because,
thankfully, children who are not abused by their caregivers are the
majority), let us consider three ordinary childhood traumas—
events that developed into trauma, rather than just fright or hurt.
Take a few moments to view things through the eyes of five-year-
old Dylan, who gets off the school bus at the wrong stop, three-
year-old Amy, who has surgery for a cleft palate, and nine-year-old
Matthew, who sees his mother break her own china dishes:

Dylan started kindergarten on Tuesday. Today is Wednesday.
He is riding the school bus home for the second time in his life. He
feels a little intimidated by the big ten-year-old sitting beside him,
he misses his mother, and he is not at all sure that he knows how to
be a school bus rider. Nearly everything during the past day and a
half has been new, and Dylan is worn out, and eager to get back to
the homey sofa in the den, and his Quack Pack videos. His mother
promised that she would be waiting for him at the bus stop, just

like yesterday. He looks expectantly out the window as the bus travels by places that look dimly familiar.

When the bus finally stops, bunches of loud, laughing, pushing children migrate hastily toward the door. The children disembark in an impenetrable tangle of thrashing heads and arms, Dylan among them, confused but earnestly striving to be a good bus rider. There are some adults by the side of the road. They greet the children, and in a matter of seconds, the bus has departed, and everyone has moved away from the bus stop.

Dylan's mother is not there. And as people walk out of sight, chattering and swinging each other's hands, no one notices that one five-year-old boy has been left standing alone.

The boy does not even think about calling after the people. He is too stunned, and besides, he does not know them. He stands right there, for a long time, hoping that his mother will appear. He looks like a tiny statue at the edge of the road, until a monstrous truck, air horn blaring, zooms by just a few feet in front of him, causing him to lurch sideways into some trees. He looks around at the wooded area, and decides he had better hide there until his mother comes.

Dylan sits down under an elm, where he is concealed from the road by a small embankment. He puts his legs out in front of him, and leans back against the tree. His new backpack, which he still has on, cushions him a bit. He stares straight ahead, and begins to tap his new sneakers together. He is scared, but he knows his mother will come soon. He sits that way for about half an hour, the length of one Quack Pack video, and then he thinks the unthinkable: maybe she is not coming. As soon as this thought occurs to him, he feels clammy all over; his stomach feels shaky, and he begins to cry. Soon, the tears have turned to desperate sobs. He cries convulsively for several minutes, until he is gasping for breath. Then, he gets an idea. He inhales as deeply as he can, stands up, and walks cautiously back to the roadside, where he looks around briefly. He calls out, "Mommy!" and then, more emphatically, "Mommy!"

Dylan is about three quarters of a mile from his home, in a nice, safe suburban neighborhood. As long as he stays out of the road, which he knows to do, he is in no physical danger. Serene middle-class houses sit at the ends of the driveways that join the street on both sides. Really, all that Dylan has to do is go up one of the driveways and knock on a door, which in all likelihood will be answered by a sympathetic adult who will quickly contact his mother. But five-year-old Dylan does not know this. In his so-far brief time on earth, he has never knocked on a strange door. He has never even gone all alone to someone else's house. And in his current panicked state, he does not even put it together that the silent houses contain people at all. The houses are only another aspect of what is impersonal and frightening all around him.

After shouting "Mommy" a few more times, he gives up and returns to his tree behind the embankment. His pants are damp in back, from the ground he sits on. He feels cold in the warm September afternoon, and he shivers. He whispers "Mommy" once, and a few more tears leak onto his cheeks. But then he is quiet. He sits quite still under the tree, as the enormity of his situation engulfs him. He is lost. His mother is gone. He will never get to talk to her again. He is never going home.

In this way, he remains for about another hour. He begins to feel that the world is very far away, and he is just a teeny speck floating somewhere in a fuzzy gray space. He wonders, in a detached sort of way, whether he is going to die now. Finally, he does not feel anything, not even cold and shivery. Still wearing his backpack, he curls up in a fetal position on the ground, and, in his mind, completely disappears from himself and his surroundings.

Another hour passes. Dylan is brought back to himself when his mother dives to her knees by the tree, and grabs him up in her arms. Some other grown-ups are there, also. Without emotion, Dylan says, "Mommy?" His mother is sobbing and jubilant at the same time, and she does not notice that Dylan is neither.

Someone drives Dylan and his mother home. They sit in the backseat, where his mother hugs and kisses him over and over, and tells him that everything is okay. Dylan does not say anything. When they get home, his mother places several emotional phone calls, and then she makes some chicken noodle soup for Dylan. When he does not eat it, she tells him once again that everything is okay. She assures him that from now on, she will pick him up at kindergarten herself. No more school bus. Then, feeling at a loss, she suggests that they sit on the cozy sofa together and watch one of his videos. She holds him close, and he watches the movie. He does not keep up a running commentary, or wiggle away to bounce on the furniture the way he usually does, but she knows that he must be exhausted, and probably still frightened. She is, too.

When the movie is over, she decides that Dylan looks pale. She hopes he has not gotten sick from lying on the damp ground, and she suggests that he go to sleep right now, though it is still early. Without protest, Dylan lets his mother put him to bed, where he resumes his fetal position.

When we imagine this event from inside Dylan's mind, we see that he is much more than tired and very scared. He is traumatized. His nascent views of the world and the people in it have been violated, and his ability to cope has been utterly overwhelmed. At the age of five, he has imagined the face of death, and has experienced the fact that one can terminate such imaginings by being dissociative. All of this without any objective danger, and though the story had a happy ending.

Now let us visit the mind of another child, three-year-old Amy, who has just had surgery.

Amy's parents love her dearly. After she was born, when the doctor said she had a cleft palate, they vowed to make the impending medical procedures as comfortable and nontraumatic as possible for their little daughter. It is now two in the morning on the day after Amy has had an operation intended to improve her speech. She is waking fully for the first time since the surgery, in a private hospital room, where both of her parents lie asleep on cots beside her bed. But it is pitch-dark in the room, and Amy does not know her parents are there, nor does she know where she is. Groggily, the last thing she remembers is going with her parents to a scary hospital, and getting a shot. She wonders whether she is now somehow at home in her bed. She starts to lift her head, but when she does, her neck hurts—a lot. She puts her arms out, and they hit hard, cold things close to her on both sides. Frightened, she jerks her arms back, and lies still. The darkness mercifully prevents her from seeing the IV needle in her left forearm.

Then she remembers what they told her about having an operation and staying in the hospital. They told her she would sleep in a bed there. But recalling this information does not help her. She is becoming more scared. Why is it so dark? Is it night? At home she has a night-light. She wants a night-light, and she wants her mother. She tries to call "Mommy," but all that comes out of her is a small, soft sound, not "Mommy" at all. And for some reason, it hurts to try.

She stops attempting to speak, and lies still again. And then the real pain starts. Quite unknown to Amy, her analgesic medication is running out. In about fifty minutes, a nurse will come into the room and administer some more painkiller; but this is going to be a long fifty minutes for Amy. The pain starts to swell up in her mouth and head so much that she cannot stand it. What is happening? Why does her head hurt so bad? Tears pool in her eyes and overflow in streams to her ears. The room is dark; she cannot see. And she is alone.

She stays as still as she can, and tries to understand. What is wrong with her? What did Mommy and Daddy say was wrong with her? Something about her mouth, her "palate," they kept saying. What is that? She cannot remember. But she remembers that she is not like other kids. There is something wrong with her. She remembers that there is something really wrong with her.

The pain gets stronger, and Amy wonders whether she is dying, like when they had to put Winston to sleep at the animal hospital. Maybe Mommy and Daddy left her here just the way they left Winston. There was something wrong with him too. She tries to call out again, but no sounds come, just more pain. By now it hurts so much that she can hardly breathe. She crawls inside her head and watches the pain. It is a bright light, and gets brighter and brighter when she looks. After a minute or two, Amy's body seems to disappear, and the only thing left is the light.

By the time the nurse arrives, right on schedule, to give a pain reliever, Amy's body temperature has dropped to ninety-six degrees. Thinking that Amy is asleep, because she is so still, the nurse quietly adds another blanket to her coverings. Then, the nurse realizes that Amy's eyes are open. Having promised Amy's mother and father that she would alert them, the nurse switches on a dim light, and gently rouses them, where they have been exhausted and asleep on their cots. Amy's parents jump up immediately. The mother sees that her little girl's face and hair are damp, and wonders in consternation whether she has been lying there crying.

Amy's mother squeezes Amy's hand and whispers in her ear, "Mommy and Daddy are here, sweetie. The operation's over. You did great. Everything's okay."

Another happy ending. Amy's loving parents soon take her home, where they continue to care for her solicitously.

She will never tell them about her fifty minutes of terror; three-year-old Amy has no words for this. And her mother and father will never coax her to tell them, because from their perspective, nothing happened.

Finally, let us imagine the inner life of nine-year-old Matthew, whose resentful and embattled parents have frequent screaming arguments with each other in their home. The fights are mainly verbal, but Matthew experiences these clashes as extremely frightening, despite the customary lack of physical violence. He worries that his family will fall apart. He wonders what will happen to him. And, as children do, he thinks that, somehow, everything must be his fault.

His mother is especially rageful and impulsive. When she gets mad, she looks like a different person. She screws up her face and clenches her fists, and appears to want to kill someone. And in fact, when she is fighting with her husband, she usually says that someday she will murder him. Each time Matthew overhears this declaration, he feels hollow and numb.

On this particular evening, Matthew's father has stomped out of the house and driven away in his car, in the middle of another loud, vicious dispute. A tearful Matthew has been hiding in his bedroom, pretending to watch television. When he hears his father leave, he tiptoes down to the kitchen to check on things. His mother is standing there, facing the kitchen sink, her hands clutching its edge. Her shoulders are heaving, and she is muttering profanities. Matthew decides to go back to his bedroom, but before he can withdraw, his mother whirls around and begins to scream the same curses at the top of her lungs. She is shaking all over. She glances around the kitchen for a moment, until her eyes settle on a large china pitcher, one of her prized possessions. While Matthew watches in horror, she grabs the pitcher and hurls it against a wall. The pitcher shatters, spraying its shards all over the floor.

Then, she notices Matthew. She says, "Hello, offspring. Watch this." And with Matthew as her stupefied witness, she yanks open the glass doors of the hutch that holds her gold-rimmed wedding china, and proceeds to snatch out all the dinner plates, one by one, hurling each against the wall, as if it were a discus. She punctuates each demolition with an epithet, such as "That maggot!" Before long, there is a wide, jagged bank of ruined china on the kitchen floor. When all the plates are gone, she sits down on the marble tiles, beside the mess she has made, and weeps.

Trembling visibly—because his mother, this inescapable adult, seems lethally out of control—Matthew gets a broom and a dustpan, and tries to restore some order. He deposits all the broken china into three large paper bags.

After a while, his mother calms down, and thanks him.

The following morning, when Matthew gets out of bed and begins to dress, he remembers unhappily that his parents had another fight last night. He thinks his father left in the middle, but he is not sure. Matthew does not remember going downstairs after he heard his father's car drive away. He has no memory of the debacle that happened in the kitchen. He believes he spent last night watching TV in his room, but perplexingly, he cannot recall what was on.

Matthew goes to school feeling depressed on account of the fight, but he will never remember the scene that overwhelmed him completely, and caused him to phase out. And his parents will never turn their attention to his psychological well-being, and ask him how he is coping with their tumultuous household. They have too much trouble of their own.

Dylan, Amy, and Matthew have gone through situations that most adults, looking on from the outside, would describe as "awful," or "so frightening," or perhaps "ugly." But for the children, these events were beyond awful; they were traumatizing. These three children were not deliberately abused, as Julia was, but their young meaning systems were violated, and their limited self-protective strategies were tested to the point of failure. However briefly, a corridor to annihilation opened up in each new soul. But neither Dylan nor Amy nor even nine-year-old Matthew will, as adults, have intelligible memories of the traumatic episodes in their lives. When they are grown, should anyone have occasion to ask them whether they were ever traumatized in childhood, they—like most of us—will answer with a confident "No, of course not."

These are illustrations of *primary trauma* occurring undetected in the lives of ordinary, nonabused children from nice neighborhoods in the developed world. Disturbing enough. But chillingly, trauma has a second, even more covert mechanism. It can affect children and adults directly, as in primary trauma, or it can function vicariously, make a long, stealthy leap from one person's mind to another person's, across space and time. *Secondary trauma*, the vicarious sort, is a term used most often by psychotherapists, to refer to the fact that a person (such as a psychotherapist) can begin to show significant symptoms of post-traumatic stress disorder merely from hearing repeated stories about the traumatic experiences of other people (such as trauma patients). Secondary trauma quietly and pervasively occurs even in the lives of those who are not psychotherapists and who do not treat trauma patients, for the simple reason that, in a world where too many children have never even slept on a mattress, extreme human misery is not far removed from any of us.

In 1993, the International Federation of Red Cross and Red Crescent Societies stated in *World Disaster Report* that in the quarter century between 1967 and 1991, disasters in various places around the world killed seven million people, and directly affected another three billion. In the same report, the Red Cross estimated that, between the end of World War II and 1991, about forty million people were killed in wars and conflicts, our perennial man-made disasters.

Indeed, viewed in cold objectivity, we are shell-shocked as an entire species.

If we travel a little away from the developed world, we find that more than one fifth of the global population still lives in extreme poverty, and life expectancy in some of the least-developed countries is forty-three years. At least one billion people now living on our planet suffer from chronic hunger, and a human child dies from malnutrition every four seconds. The World Health Organization reports that half of humanity still lacks regular access to the treatment of common diseases, and to the most basic medicines.

In terms of both space and time, we are not very far away from similar levels of human suffering, though we seldom reflect upon the fact. If the history of humanity is compared to an hour, the so-called developed world is but a few seconds old. Many of our great-grandparents, and even some of our grandparents, spent most of their lives in conditions we would consider unbearable.

Commonplace horror is only two or three generations behind us, and in places, not behind us at all. The Holocaust is a living memory. Other projects of ethnic genocide are being pursued even as these words are written.

And most of us have heard the stories, usually while we were children, and usually from people we cared about. For some, the accounts were only of the walking-to-school-five-miles-through-the-snow variety. But for others, the stories were about surviving daily hunger, or a war, or a death camp.

One of the most poignant examples of secondary trauma that I have ever known involved a woman who had seen various therapists because of a vivid nightmare. This nightmare wrecked her sleep every night, leaving her chronically sleep-deprived and exhausted. Forty-four-year-old Magda was the granddaughter of a Polish physician, whose daughter, Magda's mother, had emigrated to the United States just after World War II. When she left Europe, Magda's mother was the only surviving member of a large family that had been decimated in the camps.

Magda's father was an American physician, whom her mother had met soon after her arrival here, while he was still a student. On account of her father, Magda's own childhood and adolescence, spent in an idyllic setting in western Massachusetts, had been financially privileged; and because of her mother, she had been a gently treated and obsessively watched-over child.

"Salon appointments were always the big thing. She always had my hair done, even when I was quite little."

As an adult, Magda kept her brown hair very long, and wore it invariably in an elaborate French braid.

When I asked Magda whether she had ever been traumatized, she replied, in wholly unaccented English, "No, of course not. Nothing like that." But somehow, even given her considerable intelligence and her distinguished forebears, Magda had not lived up to her family's ambitions for her. As a child, she had wanted to be a doctor, like her father and her legendary grandfather. Instead, she had dropped out of Harvard University in her junior year, and had spent more than two decades being haunted by her nightmare, suffering intermittently from major depression, and barely getting by as a nurse's aide.

"It's the story my mother told me," she explained, sallow-faced and sad, "except it's not my mother. It's me."

"It's you? You mean it's you in the dream?"

"Yes. It's what happened to my mother, only it's happening to me. Over and over again, every night."

"Your mother told you a story about what happened to her in the war?"

"Oh yes, many times. Always the same story, about the camp."

"How old were you when she first told you this story?"

"I don't know, really. I don't remember a time when I didn't know it. I must have been really little."

"And your dream is always the same?"

"Always the same. Always just as bad. I'm with a lot of people, in some kind of a long line. I'm naked, and I'm really, really cold. Someone shoves me down to the ground, and I see that they're taking away my mother and my father. I scream 'Mother!' but someone kicks me hard. I wake up screaming. I wake up screaming every night."

"Is this exactly what your mother told you about what happened to her?"

"Yes, exactly . . . except, well, except that she was not a tiny child, and in my dream, I'm a tiny child."

"That's so terrifying. When you wake up screaming from the dream, what do you do?"

"I get up and walk around my apartment. I turn on all the lights, and I touch things. I touch my big couch and the soft draperies. I touch the numbers on my kitchen phone, all like that. I need things to bring me back to the here and now, or something. The dream is so *real*. And after I've done that for a while, I think I start to get really numb. Not frightened by the dream anymore—instead I get, well, kind of feeling-less. I wake up on the couch a lot in the mornings."

Magda was tormented by this dream every night of her life, and our progress in therapy was extremely slow.

While she was still quite young, she had made a vow never to become a mother herself. During one session, when I asked her why, she answered without hesitation that the world was just too dangerous for children.

"But you live in New England," I said, "and World War II was so long ago."

"You're right, of course," she replied. But then she looked away, and stared in silence at an empty chair across the room.

CHAPTER FOUR

Pieces of Me

*It is by no means certain that our individual personality
is the single inhabitant of these our corporeal frames . . .
We all do things both awake and asleep which surprise us.
Perhaps we have co-tenants in this house we live in.*

—Oliver Wendell Holmes

On a different day, in that same room, Julia and I sat across from each other in two wide, low leather chairs. The feeling imparted by the office we occupied was one of absolute self-containment and old-fashioned solidity, even weightiness. The ceiling in the turn-of-the-century Back Bay room was high, grand, and trimmed with mahogany, and the walls were lined with brimming hardwood bookshelves. Russet-toned oriental rugs lazed on the floor, and a pine fire murmured discreetly from inside an ornate mantle taller than a person.

Ten feet behind me, twin nine-foot hand-carved doors, now securely closed, concealed an adjacent pair of equally massive doors, also shut, to the waiting room—the famous double doors of vintage therapy rooms, designed to insure privacy, and the rarity of total silence. Fifteen feet behind my hopeful new hypnosis subject, floor-to-ceiling windows surrounded her with the pearlescent light of a Boston fog, into which the rest of the world is consumed and erased. In all, the room was a beautiful vault, in which auburn-haired Julia glowed in the ethereal white dress she had chosen specially for this occasion—and from which everything else was scrupulously banished.

Ambience has been important to hypnotists from the beginning, although settings have not always been this sedate. Working in Paris just before the Revolutionary bloodletting began, the eighteenth-century Viennese physician Franz Anton Mesmer (from whom we derive the verb "to mesmerize") placed his patients, mostly "hysterical" Parisian society ladies, in magnetic tubs filled with glass powder and iron filings. The room in which he "healed" his subjects, according to his theory of "animal magnetism," was in half-darkness, and mirror-filled. And as a commissioned glass harmonica player delivered soothing tones from behind curtains adorned with astrological symbols, Mesmer, an imposingly large individual, would enter dressed in a long purple robe and carrying an iron wand, and proceed to induce his miraculous "magnetic trance."

"*Dormez!*" he would command. (Sleep!) And Parisian high society in the Age of Reason would perform eye rolls, tremble, tingle, cry out in wonder, and swoon. Once hypnotized, Mesmer's subjects would often enter a frenzied state that resembled demonic possession, whereupon they were taken away, by Mesmer's assistants, to a mattress-lined "crisis room."

The process was believed to induce the flow of a healing magnetic fluid, thus restoring diseased bodies to well-being through magnetic harmony with the universe.

Queen Marie Antoinette was enchanted by Mesmer's activities, but in 1784, King Louis XVI, annoyed, appointed a special committee of the French Academy of Sciences to investigate his claims. This committee, which included Benjamin Franklin among its members, soon discredited Mesmer's theory entirely, proclaiming that "imagination without magnetism may produce conversions; magnetism without imagination produces nothing." His heyday at an end, Mesmer retired to the region of Europe that is now Switzerland—an outcome that may well have prevented him from losing his head quite literally—and died an impoverished unknown at the age of eighty-one. Still, Mesmer's influence has proved enduring and diverse. He has crept into our dictionary. And admirers of Mozart may recall the magnetic cure that occurs in *Così fan tutte*.

Hypnosis, then, began as a show-stopping, star-studded fraud, the spectacular invention of a gifted fanatic. Little wonder that people's reactions to hypnosis, even today, are—simultaneously—skepticism, fascination, and fear. Also, one may detect more than a hint of sexism in the origins of hypnotism, a sinister undertone that has, in fact, carried through to our own time.

Hypnosis as it is practiced today began with James Braid, working in England, who discovered in 1843 that a state of "nervous sleep" (in retrospect, a forgivable misnomer) could be induced simply by focused attention or "fixity of gaze." It was he who first referred to the process as "hypnosis," after the Greek god of sleep. And from 1845 to 1853—at just about the time ether, too, began its tenure as an anesthetic—James Esdaile, a Scottish physician working in Calcutta, performed more than three hundred painless surgeries, including amputations and cataract extractions, using only trance to control pain. And here, along with the blessed benefits, entered racism as well, for Esdaile noted in his writings that the denizens of India were simply more hypnotizable than those of Europe.

In the second half of the nineteenth century, hypnosis was reintroduced into France, most popularly by the neurologist Jean-Martin Charcot, who, among many other lasting accomplishments, was among the first to discuss systematically the concept of dissociation. Charcot attracted students from all over Europe, and was another hypnotist to realize the benefits of a dramatic setting, though his of a more credible sort. In arresting and strategically elegant demonstrations performed at Paris's medically renowned, historically gruesome La Salpêtrière, Charcot hypnotized his "hysterical" female patients for the edification of groups of students and others, who soon began to call him "the Napoleon of the neuroses." Charcot's students included Pierre Janet, Joseph Breuer, and another young Viennese physician, Sigmund Freud—although Freud, according to his own records, was never a very good hypnotist. By the turn of the twentieth century, Freud had abandoned the use of trance, in favor of the technique of free association, and later, psychoanalysis.

Charcot described how a traumatically generated *"choc nerveux"*—the result of an unbearable experience—could propel an individual into a mental state similar to the trance that might be induced by a hypnotist. Later, his student Janet proposed that overly frightening memories cannot be integrated into normal awareness, and are therefore split off from consciousness. And these pivotal insights regarding the effects of traumatic experience, inspired in large measure by the study of hypnosis, were widely accepted by the scientific community in Europe, until psychoanalysis began to gain its almost absolute hegemony, early in the twentieth century. Psychoanalysis insisted that repressed impulses and intrapsychic conflict—rather than real experience at all—constituted the only legitimate area of inquiry into the workings of the mind.

All told, hypnosis—the intentional induction of trance—with its sensational history, is both a potential curse and a great blessing. To be sure, it is subject to human ignorance and lunacy, egoism, and the subversions of prejudice. But, as well, it can be used with remarkable results by the less greedy among us, the insightful, the compassionate, the moderate.

During World War II, and in subsequent wars, Americans discovered the advantages of hypnotic debriefings in easing "combat stress." And following the late-twentieth-century rediscovery that genuine traumatic memories are clinically important, hypnosis is being used by many therapists in their work with individuals traumatized in various ways. It can be used to provide a "safe place" in which to recall past events, and even to discuss and reframe them, such that they are more tolerable, less secret and toxic to the survivor.

I regard hypnosis with caution, maybe even a little skepticism, and also with gratitude, and at certain moments, something that approaches awe. The use of trance can speed the progress of a therapy, because it enhances recall, and I studied hypnotic techniques initially for this reason. People in their thirties, forties, fifties, and older, for whom the reality of extreme trauma is twenty, thirty, forty or more years in the past, are often impatient, and rightfully so, with the lingering, life-depleting effects of those ancient events. Too often, they are close to despair, to viewing their lives as aborted attempts, as hopeless mismatches. And so, if I believe that a person is ready to deal with the past, has sufficient internal and external resources to face the extremely unsettling material that may be uncovered, I will suggest hypnosis as a part—and only a part—of our work together. Vital nonhypnotic treatment components include providing a safe *holding environment* (making certain that the therapy as a whole constitutes a caring "safe place"), *cognitive restructuring* (the therapeutic reexamination of long-standing belief systems), and *affect toleration* (teaching constructive ways to live with powerful emotions).

When using hypnosis, I remain severely cautioned, and repeatedly warn my patients, that the memories we may call forth were originally dissociated from consciousness for a very good and life-preserving reason, and for this we must retain the utmost respect. Proceed with great care. I have no magic iron wand, and ethical hypnotherapy is much more than mere theater.

Sitting across from me in the warm and vaultlike atmosphere of this present-day office, waiting to be hypnotized for the first time, Julia, of course, asked me the two questions that seem to get at the heart of the matter for most people.

She wanted to know, "Are you going to make me cackle like a chicken?"

"No, I'm not going to make you cackle like a chicken. It's a co-operative effort. You would have to *let* me make you cackle like a chicken."

"Well I'm not going to."

"Good."

And then, understandably, she wanted to know how hypnosis *works*. What was my opinion, anyway?

I said, "My opinion about hypnosis is that it's dissociative. Remember our talks about how, when something triggers you, a part of your 'self' leaves, and you go on behaving, but without self-awareness? That's when you have the sense of losing time; you wake up on a Tuesday, and then you discover it's Friday."

"Yes, of course I remember. How could I forget that?"

"I think hypnosis is like that. In the case of hypnosis, a person dissociates from . . . well, I picture it as letting go of the sentry that guards the entrance to conscious thought, the portion of your mind that you're usually aware of, which is only a very small portion because the sentry keeps it that way. You let go of the sentry, along with your conscious thoughts, and when you do that, then things going on in your mind that you're not usually aware of can get in; they can make themselves known. Sometimes they can even talk out loud."

"Oh great. So what you're saying is that you're going to make me dissociate, you're going to make me do the very thing I spend most of my life trying not to do."

"Well, first of all, I'm not going to *make* you do anything. I'd like to teach you how to do something, if you'd like to be taught. And yes, I do think you'll dissociate—but with a big difference. I can show you how to do it voluntarily instead of reflexively, the way it is now. And even better, I can teach you how to come out of the trance whenever you want to."

Julia really liked that last part. Most people do.

I asked, "Still want to go ahead with this today?"

"Yes, I think I really do," she said.

"Why don't we start, then? Just relax, and if you feel comfortable closing your eyes, that would be good."

Dutifully, Julia sank into her leather chair, and closed her eyes.

For a moment, I regarded the trusting and now-blind first communicant in front of me. In the diffused light, in her white dress, she looked as though she might ascend. And here, one more time, was my excruciating dilemma:

I was about to hypnotize Julia, toward the goal of helping her to remember more about her tortured past. Encouraging her to retrieve such memories was harrowing enough; but the real problem was this: the common but bedeviling fact that not all of our memories are true. Memory and imagination swirl around each other in the human mind, embrace and retreat from each other, and embrace again, in an intricate and mysterious dance that occurs beyond our awareness. We can have accurate memories. We can have dreams, fascinating confabulated visions. And we can have memory-dreams, things that combine the force of our actual past experience with the spellbinding creations of fancy.

Anyone who has ever been bemused by feeling that a certain memory may be real or may rather be the fleeting detail from a recent dream, and anyone who understands that a particular childhood anecdote may be her own memory or may rather have come from hearing others tell a story many times, can appreciate the potential confusion between memory and imagination.

An arresting vision, a metaphor, may in some sense contain more truth than does a hard fact. For example, if someone has been seriously abused in childhood by her Uncle Ned, she may be haunted by the image of, say, Uncle Ned scooping her up in a wheelbarrow, hauling her off to the woods near her childhood home, and burying her alive. This image carries the power of meaning, and arguably contains more truth about her past than does the lusterless fact that Uncle Ned never even owned a wheelbarrow. But this, the image, the metaphor, is not good enough, because for the most part, people in therapy (and outside of it) are explicitly looking for facts. And when people think they have found the facts, they will usually base their feelings, thoughts, and actions upon them. Should our fictitious image-maker come to believe that she was in fact buried alive, this belief will forever alter her relationship with her Uncle Ned, in ways she might not choose should she understand her "memory" to be a metaphor, something that communicates the experience of an abused child, but not something that documents specific fact.

The question of memory, and its sources, intrigued and maddened psychotherapists during the entire twentieth century, and will continue to plague us. If a person says to her therapist, "When I was little, my sister watched while I nearly drowned in the sea," is this a statement of fact, or an analyzable metaphor produced by the bottomless creativity of the "unconscious" mind? Freud asked this sort of question, and after a brief period of considering childhood trauma as a source of adult pathology, soon arrived at his inestimably influential conclusion that, no, such stories were not based upon actual past trauma, but were instead the imaginal productions of intrapsychic conflict. Dissociation was not fundamentally a reaction to life experiences, but was instead the pathological outcome of the individual's internal struggles. His theories inaugurated the larger part of a century in which psychiatry fixated upon fantasy rather than real life.

Viewed in this way, Julia, for example, would not be seen as the survivor of an abusive childhood, but rather as a "neurotic" person whose repressed infantile sexuality was creating dissociative "symptoms."

Freud, to put it succinctly, did not believe that his patients' memories were real.

Currently, with stronger interest in treatments for post-traumatic stress disorder, and with our increasing understanding that childhood trauma is heartbreakingly common, the issue of recall has heated up anew, in the form of the "false memory" debate. If a person says to her therapist, "My stepfather raped me," is this state-ment literally true? Or is it something she only imagines to have happened, because she never liked her stepfather? Or—a new one for the end of the twentieth century and the beginning of the twenty-first—does the statement have its roots in a notion that a too-zealous therapist accidentally, or even willfully, planted in the patient's mind?

Those who believe that retrieved memories are false can point to some of the most hideous cases of malpractice imaginable, in which the legal system has sometimes become involved, and in which the lives of individuals and entire families have been devas-tated, because false memories have been encouraged or even im-planted. These cases, some of them well documented, make one's blood run cold, especially if one happens to be a psychotherapist.

Those who believe that retrieved memories are true can cite re-search done at Harvard, Berkeley, UCLA, Yale, the Menninger Clinic, and other institutions, and in countries as diverse as the United States, Israel, and Australia, indicating first that trauma-genic amnesia exists, and second that memories retrieved after a period of forgetting are often quite accurate.

Opposing arguments concerning the "false-memory" issue have become polarized and strident, as people perceive—and imagine—various social, legal, and political consequences. These feared con-sequences, on one side or the other, range from wholesale cultural denial of child sexual abuse as a problem, to widespread persecu-tion of certain psychotherapists, to unprecedented changes in the legal system, to an antifeminist backlash. And, ironically, fear has gotten in the way of a more levelheaded approach to the available facts.

So what are the available facts? There are not a lot, at present, but what we do now know is crucial. We can say with certainty that the century-old tradition of memory analysis in psychotherapy does involve the risk of abuse, accidental and otherwise, particu-larly as the legal system has become involved, because about twenty percent of the general population is demonstrably "highly suggestible." On the other hand, we can say with certainty, also, that therapy is the least commonly reported trigger for recall; trauma-specific reminders and adult life crises are most frequently cited, by far, and the intrusion of new memories is often given as a reason to seek therapy in the first place.

Regarding brain activity itself, cognitive neuroscientists inform us that neuropeptides and neurotransmitters released during stress often affect memory function, acting upon the amygdala, the hippocampus, and other brain regions involved in memory. Chronic childhood abuse may result in long-term modulations in the function of these neurochemicals. Brain imaging studies indicate that childhood abuse is associated with long-term changes in declarative memory (sometimes called "explicit memory"), in the same pattern found in persons diagnosed with combat-related post-traumatic stress disorder.

In addition to knowledge gained from neuroscience, we know from sociological research conducted using early hospital records that at least some people victimized in childhood forget the documented abuse for a period of time, and later retrieve accurate memories of it.

But we know also that it is entirely possible—in fact, in some people it is easy—to suggest and instill dramatically false "memories," even easier to discuss and encourage a person's own doubts and vague suspicions such that they take on the quality of memory. Recently, even practitioners who understand the therapeutic significance of recovered memories have begun to publish warnings and guidelines, regarding the importance of outside corroboration, the tracking down of medical records, and possible witnesses, friends, relatives, old neighbors. They highlight as well the obligation to confirm symptoms that are specifically associated with previous traumatic experience (nonorganic amnesia for substantial portions of the past, conspicuous dissociative episodes in the present).

The warnings strongly emphasize the need for therapeutic neutrality, and a clear understanding on the part of the therapist of the difference between historical truth (an entirely factual account) and narrative truth (an account that may include gaps, representative stories, and metaphors, in addition to factual information). Most severely, the guidelines admonish against mixing the roles of therapeutic and forensic expert.

And so, the answer to the question of the accuracy of recovered traumatic memories is neither black nor white. The answer, like the answer to so many other important questions, is gray, and comes wrapped in many caveats and admonitions. Sometimes a recovered memory is factual. Sometimes it is, in part or in whole, a product of the imagination, or even of someone else's imagination.

But the two most compelling facts we know about this issue, forming a mandate that simply will not go away, are first, that in report after report, the "dissociative disorders" are correlated with childhood trauma, and second, that the treatment of traumatic memories is crucial to the recovery of persons with debilitating dissociative reactions. If we are to provide lasting relief for people whose dissociative behavior has crippled them, then we must deal with the slippery, political, explosive entity of *memory*. Dark corridors or not, we have to try to find our way; for if we dismiss the past as altogether and forever lost, simply because we cannot reconstruct individual histories in hour-by-hour forensic detail, then our trauma patients are lost to us, too.

What of hypnosis itself? Most brain scientists who study trance propose some alteration in *supervisory attention* during hypnosis— figuratively speaking, some at least partial deposing of the vigilant mental sentry of which I had just spoken to Julia. And hypnosis is not just a neurological phenomenon; it is also an interpersonal influence process, unavoidably. Even when they claim to be skeptical regarding hypnotism, most people *believe* in it ("whatever 'it' is," as Julia had once quipped), such that the hypnotist herself wields more power than she may wish to have. Remarks and suggestions made by the hypnotist are often accepted by the hypnotic subject as uncritically as charged, far-rippling spatters of rain are received by a very calm lake.

I have always felt somewhat daunted when beginning a course of hypnosis with someone, because it is so powerful, and also because it has the potential to uncover material that the subject's mind has insistently kept under wraps, sometimes for decades. Still staring at the white-clad Julia, I took one long, deep breath, and focused on the job at hand. Apart from the fire rustling softly in the hearth, there was utter silence in the room, until I said—

"That's good. You can just relax."

Cooperatively, Julia let her head loll slightly forward, and a lock of her hair fell over her right eye.

"Just relax and listen to the sound of my voice. That's all you have to do. For just a little while, that's all you have to do. Just listen to the sound of my voice. Everything else is far, far away. Only the sound of my voice is here. For just a little while, you can relax, and just listen to the sound of my voice."

I let four or five beats go by, and then continued. My words became slow, repetitive, and hazily enigmatic:

"From time to time, while you're listening to the sound of my voice, there may be other noises. Maybe a car will go by. Maybe the telephone will ring, or maybe there will be the sound of children playing outside the window. And that's perfectly okay. It just doesn't matter. You can notice those noises, and maybe they will sound softer than they usually do, or maybe they will sound more distinct than they usually do. Either way, it just doesn't matter. You can hear the noises, and just let them go by. Just let them go by, because for just a little while, all that really matters is the sound of my voice as I talk to you. All that really matters is the sound of my voice. You can let go of everything else. It feels so good, just to let go of everything else."

Julia's chin reached her chest. With a deep sigh, she sleepily raised her hands from her lap and let them rest on the arms of her chair.

"Very good," I continued. "Just relax. Get as comfortable as you can, and just relax.

"Sometimes while you're just relaxing, you may find that thoughts come into your head, thoughts about this and that, thoughts that come into your head. And that's perfectly okay. That's perfectly normal. You can let thoughts drift into your head. They can be there for a little while, and then you can let them drift out again, like puffy white clouds drifting across a beautiful blue sky. Your thoughts are like the clouds. Just like the clouds, they drift into view. Who knows why? They just drift into the sky. They're there for a little while, and then after a little while, they drift away again. They're gone, all by themselves."

Julia was very relaxed now. Her breathing was deep and even.

I let a few more beats go by, and then went on:

"Very good. You're doing very well. And now while you're very relaxed, if it's okay with you, I'm going to have you relax all the parts of your body just a little bit more. You can always become just a little bit more relaxed.

"I'd like you to start by allowing your mind to focus on the feelings in your hands. Just relax, and notice how your hands feel as they rest against the arms of the chair. Notice how the leather feels against your skin, smooth and nice.

"And now, if it's okay, I'd like you to imagine that a wonderful sense of deep relaxation and calm is spreading through your hands. Deep relaxation has flowed into your hands, into your palms and all the way out to the tips of your fingers. And now both hands are very calm, very loose and limp. Relaxed.

"And now I'd like you to imagine that this wonderful feeling of relaxation is beginning to spread. It's beginning to spread and travel up through your wrists, and into your forearms. It's moving from your forearms, through your elbows, and up into your upper arms. And now both of your arms are very, very relaxed, very loose and limp."

Julia sighed, and her shoulders drooped.

I continued, soothingly, to remark upon the progress of the welcome sense of relaxation, through her shoulders, up to the back of her neck, across her scalp, down over her face, and deep into her lungs.

"You feel so good. Your breathing is easy and calm, so easy and calm. And now the relaxation is flowing into your stomach. So, your whole upper body is relaxed, relaxed and very calm.

"The relaxation is moving now, down into your legs. Your upper legs feel calm and relaxed. And now it's moving through your knees, and down into your lower legs, and now both of your legs are very, very loose, very calm and relaxed. You feel the relaxation moving down through your ankles and into your feet, across the bottoms of your feet, and all the way out to the tips of your toes. Very loose. Very, very calm and relaxed."

At that instant, in the silent room, an ember in the hearth snapped like a popgun—*crack!* My eyes widened, but Julia neither moved nor altered her deep, even breathing.

"Julia, can you hear me?" I questioned.

For a moment, there was only silence; but then, from somewhere behind the auburn hair that now obscured the right half of her lowered face, came an all but inaudible "Mmm."

"Good. Very good," I said. "And now, while you're very relaxed, I'm going to count backward, very slowly, from ten down to one. And when I reach 'one,' you'll be deeply in a trance, very calm and relaxed and comfortable, and deeply in a trance.

"Starting with ten . . ."

I allowed a full twenty seconds to pass.

"Nine . . ."

I counted backward at an exquisitely slow pace, noting the numbers on my fingers so as not to lose count. When I reached "one," I questioned Julia a second time. "Can you hear me?"

"Mmm," she murmured again.

And there was Julia, dressed in white, slumped unselfconsciously in her chair. Her colorful head flagged peacefully, and her breathing was rhythmic and slow, as if she were in a profound sleep.

With most willing and cooperative subjects, and in the right setting, an experienced hypnotist can induce trance just this easily, although some people reach deeper levels of initial trance than others. Over time, as Julia and I repeated this process in many sessions, she herself would plumb deeper levels. In addition, she would enter trance more and more readily, becoming both the hypnotized and the hypnotist. Eventually, I would have only to say that we were about to begin, or perhaps to count backward from ten down to one, and an experienced Julia would independently place herself in a deep trance, needing only a few moments to accomplish the task.

But now we were going to make only a superficial first expedition into the parts of Julia's mind that were normally unvisited.

"Good. Very good," I said again. "And now, if it's okay with you, I'd like you to take a little trip inside your mind, a little trip to somewhere else, without really having to go anywhere at all. You can use your mind like a wonderful ship that will carry you wherever you want to go, and then bring you back here when you want to come back. A wonderful ship. Easy and light. And you don't even have to leave your chair.

"There's a chair. You're sitting in a chair. Can you feel the chair, Julia?"

There was a pause, and then she said, "Mmm."

She wiggled her fingers on the arms of the chair, and then a little less softly, said, "Yeah. Yeah. Chair."

My words were beyond enigmatic now; they were plainly nonsensical, not a message for the analytical part of Julia's mind, but for some other part.

"Floating in your chair," I said. "Floating and floating, to another time and another place. Floating and floating, so gently. Maybe you'll go to a place where you've been recently. Or maybe you'll float back and back, and your chair will be in a place you were long, long ago. There have been so many chairs, so many times to sit in a chair, and you're floating back to one of those. You're somewhere else, and sitting in a chair. When your chair stops floating, you will find you're somewhere else. So many pictures, so many times, but after a little while, the chair will stop, and you'll know where you are.

"You're sitting in a chair. You sit, and you know you're somewhere. Somewhere, one special place. Do you know what place you're in?"

Silence from Julia.

"Julia," I continued, "are you sitting in a chair?"

More silence, and then softly but distinctly, "Yes. Yes, in a chair."

"Where is your chair, Julia?"

"I'm not sure," she answered; and then after a moment, she continued, "I'm not really sure, but I think I know. I think I know. Is that okay?"

"It's okay, Julia. Everything's okay. Where do you think you are? What kind of chair?"

"Hard chair," she said. "Wooden chair." And then, "Can't put my arms on the table!"

In an abrupt movement, she slipped her arms off the leather armrests, and clasped her hands rigidly in her lap.

"Can't put your arms on the table?" I echoed.

"No. Not polite. Rude to put your arms on the table."

"So, is it a table for eating?"

"Yes. A table for eating. I think I'm going to be eating my lunch."

"Your lunch. I see." To evoke a visual detail, I asked, "What color are the plates?"

"The plates? Hmm. The plates are white. White. They're paper plates. I always got the paper plates at lunch. The ones with the little waves around the edge."

To myself, I noted that Julia's language ("I always got the paper plates at lunch") was not that of an especially deep trance; she was still speaking to me in the present, about something she remembered from the past, rather than reliving an experience in its immediacy. But that was okay. We had only just started.

I wondered whether I could deepen her trance a bit by suggesting another sensory detail. I asked, "Can you feel the wavy edges of the plates with your fingers?"

Julia unclenched her fingers, lifted her right hand, and moved it in a small circle twice. Her eyes still closed, she raised her head for the first time since the induction had begun, and smiled. Her blind smile was luminous.

"I feel them!" she said. "They're smooth and bumpy at the same time."

"Smooth and bumpy at the same time," I reflected back to her. "That's great. Are you hungry?"

"Hungry? Yes, hungry. I'm having lunch."

"You're having lunch. What are you having?"

There was a pause, and then Julia, her eyes still closed, said, "Hot dogs. I'm having hot dogs."

"Hot dogs. Do you like hot dogs?"

"Yes, yes, I like hot dogs. They're good."

"I'm glad you like them. Can you smell the hot dogs?"

There was another pause, and then she said in an excited tone, "Yes! Yes! I can smell them!"

There was a longer pause, during which Julia's face lost its excitement and began to register distress. After another moment, she wrinkled her nose in an expression painful to view.

"What's happening, Julia?" I asked.

"She says I have to have *that* on my hot dog. I don't want it!"

"She says you have to have it? What is it?"

"I don't want it! I don't want it! I want a plain hot dog!"

Julia began to shake her head violently back and forth. "No, no, *no*!" she said.

This little drama did not sound like child abuse per se, but it did seem distressing, and I was concerned that Julia's first experience with hypnosis might put her off the procedure. I decided it was time to end the trance.

"Julia," I said, and then a little more insistently, "Julia!"

She stopped shaking her head.

"Julia, can you hear the sound of my voice?"

After a moment in which she was quite still, she said, "Yes."

"Good. That's very good. If it's okay with you, I'd like you to come back to the chair in my office now, back to the present. Can you do that?"

"Uh-huh." She nodded her head.

"Okay. That's good. All you have to do is just listen to the sound of my voice. All you have to do is just listen. And now I'm going to count from one to five, and when I reach 'five,' you're going to be out of the trance, alert, but still calm and relaxed . . . starting with one . . . two . . . three . . . You can start to open your eyes now . . . four . . . ," and then firmly, "five."

On "three," Julia's eyes began to flutter. When I reached "five," her eyes were completely open. Her hands were loose in her lap, her face was relaxed, and she looked directly at me.

She was silent. The fire rustled.

After a few seconds, I said, "Hi. How are you?"

"I'm fine," she replied. "I feel refreshed, as if I'd been asleep for a really long time. How long was I out?"

"Oh, about half an hour, start to finish."

"That's all? Really?"

"Really."

"That was amazing," she said. "Do you know, I could actually smell that sauerkraut. I could actually *smell* it, as if it had been right under my nose, right here in this room."

"What sauerkraut?" I asked.

"The sauerkraut she made me put on my hot dog. I hated that stuff, despised it."

"Who made you put it on your hot dog?"

"She did, I mean, my mother. Wow! I could *smell* it. This hypnosis stuff is amazing. Do people always get such real sensations?"

"You did extremely well. Do you feel okay now?"

"I'm fine," she said with a big smile. She stretched her arms expansively, and appeared almost euphoric at having completed her first hypnosis session. Whatever negative emotion she had been experiencing in the trance was seemingly gone.

"When you were smelling the sauerkraut, were you frightened?" I inquired.

"Frightened? No, not frightened. Just really upset, unhappy."

"Is the upset gone now?"

"Yes, gone. I actually feel really good, as if I'd just had a nice, long sleep. I can't believe how real that stuff smelled. Vinegar! Pew!"

She pinched her nose.

After a few more minutes of debriefing, our therapy hour was over. Having satisfied myself that she was in a condition to resume her day safely, I let her go. I opened the double doors for her, and she walked out into the waiting room, her step lighthearted.

She was not always to feel so untroubled after hypnosis. After ten or eleven sessions, Julia's trances grew deep, until finally they were so profound that, had our task been to induce hypnotic analgesia, we could have done so well enough to get her through minor surgery. As Julia's experience with hypnosis increased, I began to allow her to remain in trance for longer intervals, and her memories became intensely real and sometimes terrifying. Out of trance again, Julia would no longer be frightened, but often she would be disturbed and almost unbearably saddened by the images that had just been present to her.

After three months in which Julia had hypnotic sessions once or twice a week, she announced that she would make a ten-day trip back to Los Angeles, where she had spent her childhood, to visit old neighborhoods, speak with two of her aunts, an uncle, and some former friends, and maybe even try to find the pediatrician she had been taken to a few times. The alarming memories she was retrieving, and the personal narrative of abuse they implied, compelled her to find out more about a past she had forgotten until now.

She had no siblings, and her parents had both died when she was in college, first her mother, suddenly from pancreatic cancer, and then her father, from a cirrhotic liver.

"I remember how horrible it was when they died," she had told me once. "Not because of the grief—just the opposite. I didn't feel anything. They were my parents—I mean they were my *parents*—and they died of these *hideous* diseases, and I just felt nothing. I was coldhearted. I was so coldhearted. It was shameful. . . . I'm awful. I must be truly, truly awful."

Julia was, and remains, inconsolable on this point. She will always insist that there is something very wrong with *her* that she felt nothing when her own parents died.

"I know for sure that I went to both of the funerals, but I don't remember even being at my mother's. I remember my father's a little, I guess. And I do remember the last time I saw him alive. He was in a wheelchair, old, he looked so old. He actually wanted to hold my hand, but I wouldn't . . . and he sang to me. He *sang* to me!"

She shuddered.

"He sang some of that old Beatles song about Julia. '*Ju-lee-ah! Seashell eyes. . . .* ' That one. Made my flesh crawl. Nauseous. Just got out of there as quick as I could. I went back to school."

And so Julia would have to attempt to piece some things together from the recollections, impressions, and reluctant suspicions of less immediate witnesses than her parents, who almost certainly would have kept their secrets, even had they been alive.

When she returned from Los Angeles, she described her detective project as far and away the hardest thing she had ever done. But, for Julia, the work was worth it. Her memories during hypnosis and otherwise (for by this time, she had begun to recover fragments of memory at odd moments outside of therapy), combined with the small but pointed collection of corroborating reports she had gathered in California, allowed us to clarify some portions of Julia's murky childhood.

Just after her trip, Julia raised the natural question, "How much do I have to remember in order to get better? Do I have to remember everything? When I think about it, there's so much I still don't know. I've remembered a few things, but not my whole childhood, not even close."

I have been questioned in this way many times, and my answer is always the same. No human being whatsoever, possessed of no matter how brilliant a memory, and no matter how urgent a motivation, will ever remember every single day of her past, or even every single important event. And so it is fortunate that, to recover from trauma, a person must open only a few doors, must shed some light on just a few significant occurrences, enough to construct a personal narrative, a comprehensible life story that is incomplete in its details, but meaningful in its broader themes and issues.

While answering her question, I offered Julia, the accomplished filmmaker, a question of my own: "If you were making a movie about an abused child, how many graphic scenes of abuse would you have to show on the screen to make the audience understand that the child was being abused?"

Without hesitation, Julia replied, "Only one really. Two if you wanted to hammer them over the head with the concept."

"Exactly," I said.

"Yes, well, I see what you're getting at, but I think I need to be hammered over the head quite a lot in this case."

"Okay, deal. You'll have more than two—but less than everything. You'll have several clear memories, and a lot of sensory flashes that will feel like particles of memory—smells, pictures, sounds," I said. "And now, let me ask you another strange question."

"Sure," she said, giving me a quizzical look.

"If I somehow possessed a set of videotapes that contained all the most significant events of your childhood, in their entirety, would you want to see them?"

"Absolutely. Right this very second."

"But why? Don't you think some of the tapes would be frightening and sad?"

"Most of them, yes. But if I could see them, then I could have them in my brain like regular memories—horrible memories, yes, but *regular* memories, not sinister little ghosts in my head that pop out of some part of me I don't even know, and take the rest of me away. Do you know what I mean?"

"I think so," I said. "If you have to remember, you'd rather do it in the front of your brain, not the back."

"Sort of. Yes, I guess so. I mean, the front of my brain is the part that can actually cope with things, here in the present, where I'm trying to live *now*, right?"

"Right. So as we go along, you'll make a few regular memories—not hundreds, but enough to pull all of you into your present life, and keep you there."

She thought about this for a second, and then asked, "So, what else do you think is in the back of my brain? What else am I going to find?"

"I don't know," I replied, taken aback. "If I knew that, I'd just tell you, Julia. I wouldn't put you through all this."

"Just checking," she said, and grinned.

And through Julia's brave efforts, in therapy, in hypnosis, in Los Angeles, we finally discovered a little—enough—about a young girl named Julia.

Julia's mother and father liked to play "games." One of the first traumatic memories Julia recovered under hypnosis was of a time when she was about four. ("I'm not in kindergarten yet. I'm at home with her, and he's at work.") Her mother announced that they were going to play a game of hide-and-seek.

"I'll close my eyes and count all the way to a hundred. You hide, and if I can't find you, you win. But if I do find you, then I'm going to cut off your thumbs with this knife Daddy uses to cut up chicken. No more thumbs to suck on like a big baby."

She showed Julia a knife and began to count.

"I don't know what a hundred is," the grown-up Julia said in a tiny, childlike voice in that hypnosis session in my office.

But of course little Julia had not said that out loud at the time. She simply fled in terror and searched pathetically for a place to hide. In a typically childlike strategy, she ended up in her own bedroom closet, shutting the door as well as she could from the inside. While she stood crying silently in the dark, her mother intoned all the way to "ninety-nine, one hundred," and then took an agonizingly slow tour through the house, calling out, "Mommy's gonna get you. Mommy's gonna win." No doubt guessing that Julia would have fled to her own room, the mother entered that room last, finally inching open the closet door and whispering, "Gotcha!"

Julia's parents were educated, upper-middle-class people who cared excessively about what the neighbors thought. Visible evidence of child abuse would have been unacceptable. This mother, in actuality, was not about to cut off any digits. But four-year-old Julia did not know that. She squeezed her thumbs inside her other fingers and wept so hard that she began to gag, while her mother restrained her on the closet floor, displayed the knife, and described, as if considering them, the various ways a person might go about cutting off thumbs.

In the end, the mother made a small cut at the base of one thumb, just enough to draw blood, and after making sure that Julia had seen the blood, she let the child go. Julia scrambled back into a corner of her closet and, still squeezing her thumbs, collapsed onto the floor, where her mother left her.

The mother's parting words, remembered by Julia with the particularity that people sometimes exhibit under hypnosis, were, "Now you just think about it."

When Julia's father was home, her mother showed somewhat less of her physically violent side. The "games" became more psychological and sexual. The father's favorite was an extremely abusive ritual he called "little coach," in which Julia was forced to lie in bed with her parents while they had sex. Since her father did not threaten to inflict physical injuries, Julia made one attempt, when she was still very little, to enlist his aid in dealing with her mother's violence. She showed him some bruises under her sleeves, and asked him whether he could "tell Mommy to stop doing stuff like that."

"Mommy likes to kid around sometimes," he said. "It's no big deal. You'll live."

Psychology has never adequately addressed the question of why one person will look at a vulnerable being and feel compassion, while another person will look at such a being and behave like a predator, or a sadist. The question is especially riveting when it refers to people like Julia's parents, since most mothers and fathers involuntarily experience a huge biologically prepared sense of attachment to their own offspring, paired with a commanding instinct to nurture and protect. The idea that a mother might intentionally set about to injure and humiliate her own child, might behave like Julia's mother did, is incomprehensible. And yet it happens. We read it in the papers all the time, hear about it in the news, and we are incredulous, revolted. I am appalled, still, when I read the stories, though I encounter similar ones constantly in my work, and I can assure you that hearing the stories, done without the intellectually airtight rationales of the past century, never stops being painful.

The explanation given, when considering an abusive parent, is often unconscious "identification with the aggressor." In other words, a violently abusive parent like Julia's mother is the product of parents who violently abused her, and so on back through many generations: abuse as the product of abuse as the product of abuse, and so on, like links in a chain. This is, in a sense, an unconscious and perverse version of the tactic, "If you can't beat 'em, join 'em." The helpless one, for her psychological survival while she is open to attack, "identifies" with the powerful ones, and thus endures her childhood. And when she has children of her own, the chain will continue, for the once-helpless child, now a "powerful" adult, can—and does—turn the tables at last.

The problem with this answer is that sometimes the chain gets broken. Sometimes, a person who has been abused by her parents will vow to herself that the buck stops here—and keep her vow. Consciously, vigilantly, she raises children who are genuinely cherished, nurtured, and protected—no matter how confused, depressed, and anxious she may be herself. I have known many such parents. They shine.

I cannot account for this psychologically, and no one else has ever explained it to my satisfaction. Perhaps there are intervening factors, currently mysterious, that make the difference. Or—and this thought sustains me sometimes—perhaps some special children are simply unwilling, or unable, to identify with an "aggressor" in the first place.

Two weeks after Julia's return from Los Angeles, on an unaccountably hot spring day in Boston, Julia arrived at my office for her twenty-first hypnosis session, the first hypnosis hour since her trip. For two weeks, we had spent our time in waking discussions of what she had learned on the other side of the continent, in the secret-bearing neighborhoods of her childhood. Now she was about to enter a voluntary trance again, after a break of, altogether, nearly a month. Given the intensity of our previous hypnosis sessions, the space of four weeks felt substantial.

The large windows behind Julia's chair were open, and a breeze that felt almost tropical inspirited my Boston office, dancing against the cathedral ceiling, and circling back down. Papers fluttered on a mahogany desk in the corner of the room, and as she sat facing me, Julia's hair lifted and capered around her face. Absentmindedly, she tried several times to anchor her hair behind her ears, with fleeting success. She had taken the day off from work, and was dressed in blue jeans, a sleeveless purple T-shirt, and of course, her amethyst jewelry.

By all appearances, her mood was light. Referring to the surrealistic weather, she said, "I think I must have brought southern California back with me."

"Is that a psychological statement?" I asked with a smile.

She laughed.

"Isn't everything?" she replied. And then she said, a little more seriously, "We're doing hypnosis today, right?"

"If you still want to."

"Yes, I want to. Do you think I'll remember how, after all this time?"

"Well, let's find out."

I counted backward, slowly, from ten down to one, and with no difficulty at all, Julia fell into a deep trance. Untended now, her hair blew about her as if it were weightless.

After a moment, I inquired, "Where are you today, Julia?"

Usually, she would reply right away to this question, if only to say, "I'm not sure yet." But this time there was only silence.

I decided to wait, and did so for a full three minutes by my watch. Julia was entirely still.

I said again, "Julia, where are you today?"

At this, eyes still closed, she removed an intricate amethyst bracelet from her right wrist, and began to play with it, twisting it carelessly, and then stretching the band hard enough that I feared it might come apart.

"That's a nice bracelet, Julia. Don't break it." I said.

"It's real pretty. She lets me play with it, you know. She got it at this big old building called the Jewels Building."

"You mean the Jewelers' Building?" I asked.

"Yeah, yeah! That's where she got it. Isn't it pretty? It's purple!" She stretched the bracelet again.

"It's very pretty. But who is 'she'?" I thought you bought the bracelet yourself."

"No, I didn't do that. Julia did," she said.

"Julia did. So, I'm not speaking with Julia?"

"No, silly. Do I sound like Julia?"

"Yes, you do." Or to be more accurate, she sounded like Julia attempting, without much success, to imitate a child's voice and language.

"Well, I'm not. You're silly." She giggled.

"Oh," I said. "Then who are you?"

"Amelia."

"Your name is Amelia?"

"Ah-*meel*-ya!" Julia enunciated happily.

"Hello, Amelia. How are you?"

"Good! I get to play with these pretty jewels." She was still twisting and stretching the bracelet.

"Are you a child, Amelia?"

"Course I am, silly. What did you think?"

"Well, I've never met you before, so I didn't know. How old are you?"

"Hmm. Well, I'm five. Like this." Julia held up the five fingers of her left hand. She continued in a singsong voice, "And *I* know who *you* are."

"Really? Who am I?"

"You're Martha." She pronounced the *th* with difficulty. "You're the doctor lady she always talks to."

Anywhere other than a therapist's office, this apparent transformation would have come across as bad acting, like someone with no talent playing the part of a small girl in a school play. I think that an uninitiated observer, someone who did not know that Julia was in a trance, might well have rolled his eyes and ordered her to come off it.

In the safe, soft-spoken atmosphere of therapy, sometimes people slip into what can rightfully be called an hypnotic trance even when the therapist is not intentionally attempting an hypnotic induction. Most of the time, I believe these moments pass unnoticed by both parties, and I think that gifted therapists, even when they do not consider hypnosis to be a part of their practice, often accidentally hypnotize people, by their soothing and accepting demeanor, combined perhaps with the therapy-specific pull for unconscious material. These unintended, and often unlabeled interludes can be among the most revealing and helpful of the therapeutic process.

But when a dissociated ego state, like "Amelia," speaks during one of them, these episodes can feel breathtakingly out of place. They can give the observer—the therapist, hypnotically intent in her focus upon the patient—a brief, unbidden physiological rush, like being out in the open when marble-sized hail begins to fall from a steamy August sky, and then just as suddenly stops.

The first time (to my awareness) that I encountered this circumstance was when I was a doctoral student, and a fledgling, poignantly conscientious student therapist in a counseling center. I had all the anxieties of a newcomer to anything important, but of course the very nature of the situation dictated that I reveal none of them. Everyone knows that good therapists are wise, perfectly competent, and preternaturally calm.

And I, like most of my colleagues at that point in time, had never heard of anything called a "dissociated ego state," or a "trauma-related dissociative episode."

For several weeks, I had been treating an eighteen-year-old, a straight-A high school senior, who had come to the exceedingly low-cost counseling center on her own, without her parents' knowledge, because her mother and father had "forced" her to have an early-term abortion, and she was "so depressed I can't even get myself to study anymore."

I recall that on this particular day, I was wearing a new and rather expensive taupe-colored wool suit that had been purchased for me by my own endlessly supportive and noncoercive mother, and shipped up from North Carolina to her daughter, the brand-new therapist. Most of the time, when I was not at the counseling center, I still wore jeans and sweatshirts, like any other callow twenty-two-year-old graduate student. For I was, as it happened, a meager four years older than the wounded teenager who gazed at me with such daunting respect.

Wearing a black sweatshirt and blue jeans, she sat before me in one of the eight-by-eight drywall cubicles reserved as "session rooms" by the bargain-basement counseling center. The space was furnished with two metal chairs, a peeling Formica desk, a most unsubtle twenty-dollar tape recorder, and a lopsided table lamp, meant to replace the glare of the fluorescent lighting in the drop ceiling. As I recall, a poster of fluttering pigeons in St. Mark's Square was tacked incongruously to one of the four beige walls.

We two very young women were having another conversation about the shame and grief she was experiencing around the issue of her unwanted pregnancy, and the ending of that pregnancy at an abortion clinic, which facility had released to me a succinct and un-helpful medical report about my patient's "unremarkable" first-trimester termination. Several times during the preceding weeks, she had described, in almost obsessive detail, being driven to the clinic by her silent mother and her mother's friend, the intake process, what the doctor had told her just before the procedure, the procedure itself, and the knee-hugging waves of physical agony that no one had told her about, when the Demerol wore off.

I remember that, like Julia, she had intensely blue eyes, remem-ber also that her descriptions of the medical procedure, and of the pain, made my own abdomen ache.

On this afternoon she was saying, as she had already said to me two or three times in previous meetings, "I feel like such a whore." (In point of fact, the unfortunate young woman had engaged in sexual intercourse exactly once.) "And I feel like a murderer. If only I hadn't gotten pregnant . . . but if I had to get pregnant, I think I really wanted to keep the baby. I think it really deserved to live."

She was crying softly, appropriately. She was making eye contact with me, and speaking in a sad-but-normal conversational tone. And still in the same manner, without skipping a beat, and without changing her expression or losing eye contact, she continued, "I hope they never arrest me."

"Arrest you?"

She did not seem to hear the query. She went on, in the same quietly sniffling, conversational way—but I noticed that now she was looking past me, at one of the blank walls—"She was so beautiful and tiny. I named her Gina-Marie. I dressed her all up in a little white dress, and then I got a knife and I killed her. I cut her up into pieces. Poor little baby. There was so much blood! I really didn't know there was that much blood in the whole world." And then she looked back at me and said, again without skipping a beat or altering her tone, "Our time must be almost over now." She mopped her eyes with her fingers. "Can I come back next Monday?"

In later sessions, on a wing and a prayer, I would talk with her about the profundity of her sense of guilt, and about how perhaps a part of her felt so reprehensible that it believed she was literally a murderer. But at that moment, I did nothing. I was too stunned even to be able to react. I said, "Yes, of course. I'll see you next Monday," and I let her go.

I remember there was a small mound-shaped white-noise generator just inside the door, put there in a partially successful attempt to mask the voices of passersby in the corridor outside. It whooshed dutifully from its place on the floor, and after she left, I sat in my metal chair and stared down at it for a long time, before I could manage the aplomb to get up and navigate to my next appointment, trustingly waiting for me in the counseling center's front office.

I treated the aggrieved young woman for an additional ten months, until she left for college, and I never again heard from the "murderer." I think that, to a certain degree, I eventually began to feel I had imagined the event, or perhaps misunderstood. And I can certainly comprehend how other people, not therapists, assume that they have an overactive imagination, or have probably misinterpreted, when they are exposed to similar events in the real world. In a contest among, as the only alternatives, "She's completely insane," or "I'm completely insane," or "I must have misunderstood," this third explanation—the comfort of believing that there has been some correctable misunderstanding—is going to win, hands down. This is true especially since most ego state intrusions are less blatant, more equivocal to begin with, than Julia's, or than the one that served as my initiation.

But as the years passed, years of conducting therapy, which I (like so many of my colleagues who also see trauma survivors) soon began to combine intentionally with the study and use of formal hypnotic techniques, I encountered dissociated ego states in apparently single-identity individuals so often that I ceased to react to these occurrences as if they were startling, or even unusual. In fact, I now see them as very close to routine. I am no longer taken aback or frightened—nor am I tempted to tell anyone, in therapy or in the real world, to come off it.

I continued my exchange with "Amelia," encouraging her:

"I'm the doctor lady Julia always talks to?"

"Yeah. I wanted to talk to you, too."

"You wanted to talk to me? How come?"

"Well, I'm only five, you know. I'm kind of lonely, sort of. I wish somebody would take care of me. You seem kind of nice."

"Thank you."

"Welcome."

"Does Julia take care of you?" I asked.

"She doesn't know about *me*, silly."

"Julia doesn't know about you?"

"Course not! Well . . . I guess she will now."

Through all of this, Julia's eyes remained closed, and her face was calm. Her tone of voice was vaguely more childlike than usual, higher pitched; still, she sounded more like a woman in her thirties than a five-year-old. Only her hands were completely a child's, as they recklessly played with an adult's expensive bracelet.

I said, "You mean Julia will know about you now because you've talked to me?"

"Yeah."

Abruptly, Julia's hands, along with the jewelry, fell into her lap and were still. She was silent, and there was no further movement, except for the strands of red hair floating around her impassive face, in the over-warm breeze from the windows.

"Amelia?" I prompted.

"No," came the brusque reply. There was silence for another thirty seconds, and then, "She'd ruin that bracelet, you know."

"Who would ruin the bracelet?"

"Amelia. She's cute, but she's only a kid. I told her to put it down."

Julia's voice had lost its slightly childlike character, and was now that of an annoyed adult, cynical and somewhat nasal.

"Is that you, Julia?" I asked.

"Hell no," she answered. There was another pause, and then she said, "So Doc, you really gonna help her, or what?"

"Am I really going to help whom? Julia?"

"Of course Julia. Who do you think I'm talking about? Nancy Reagan, maybe?"

Again, the sense of bad acting. Poor, dignified Julia. When she came out of this particular trance, she would be mortified.

"I certainly want to help Julia. Who are you?"

"You'd really like to know that, wouldn't you?"

"You don't have to tell me," I said.

"Yeah, you're cagey. My name is Kate, all right?"

"Hello, Kate. Do you have something to tell me?"

"Why would I have something to tell you?"

"Well, you've never spoken before, and I thought . . ."

"Yeah," she interrupted. "You thought, you thought. All right, well, I guess, since the kid let the goddamn cat out of the bag anyway, I just wanted to tell you that you better help Julia."

"I'm trying to help Julia, you have my word. Do you help her?"

"Do I really need to answer that?"

"You mean the answer is obvious?"

"Yeah."

"So I guess it's safe to say that you help Julia. When did you get your name, Kate?"

"Well, she needed *someone*, now didn't she? So she got me, Kate. They were beating up on her pretty good. She needed someone to help her forget and get out. She needed to get out, man! Put it all behind her, you know? And so I helped her do it. She was seventeen, actually, when she got me. She already had the kid."

"You mean she already had Amelia?"

"Yeah. She needed the kid too. They couldn't beat up on *her*. Nobody even knew she was there. Still don't." She chuckled, her face suddenly breaking from neutrality, becoming amused.

"So, you *protect* Julia?" I asked.

"Damn straight. I'm a black belt. And I'm watching *you*, Doc. You better stay nice."

"I intend to."

"Well, you better."

I looked at my watch, and realized there were only thirty more minutes in the therapy hour. And I knew that on this occasion, when Julia came out of her trance, she would be in shock at her own behavior. I appealed to "Kate":

"Kate, do you suppose I could have Julia back? We don't have much time left to talk, and you know Julia's going to be confused about you and Amelia."

"Yeah, she'll be pretty freaked. I'll go."

All at once, Julia's face was expressionless again. I performed my customary wake-up count from one to five, and Julia's eyes flickered open.

She was dumbfounded and appalled. I believe she would have been less astonished if a spaceship had flown in through my office window, and tiny green aliens had disembarked in front of her.

She pressed her fists against her eyes, as if trying to blot something out.

"Oh my god!" she exclaimed, as if to herself. "What was *that*? What was *that*?"

"Julia, Julia," I said, trying to get her attention. "Let's talk a little about what just happened."

"I knew I was crazy, but I didn't think I was a lunatic!"

Convincing someone who has just had such an hypnotic experience that it is not horribly unusual, and that she is not headed straight to the asylum, is difficult, perhaps impossible. But I did the best I could for Julia. I knew I would have to repeat and repeat in weeks to come, because nearly all the information I had to give her would rebound against the high-frequency barrier of her distress today, and be lost to her.

"You're not a lunatic, Julia."

"So how do you explain what just happened?"

I told her that she had experienced two dissociated ego states, and that for trauma patients in deep trance to have such episodes is not unusual. A dissociated ego state is a personality formation, or a constellation of traits and behavior patterns, of whose existence a "conscious" individual is usually unaware. A person's dissociated ego state may proclaim a proper name for itself ("Amelia," "Kate"), may be nameless, or may announce its presence with labels such as "the little one," or "the angry one," or "the sad one," or "someone with a message."

At any given point, the brain function we think of as the light of "consciousness" is capable of illuminating only a minute fraction of total brain activity, a bare inkling or two of what is really going on in our brilliant, multiplex, infuriating minds. And so for most people, the notion that an individual's brain, possibly even one's own brain, could harbor entities such as "someone with a message" or "Kate" seems the stuff of science fiction. But in reality, the human brain is more than capable of developing and housing these "extra" ego formations.

Though we do not enjoy regarding ourselves so prosaically, when all is said and done, our brains are about survival. And if rigidly compartmentalizing our selves in order to cope with the overwhelming exigencies of chronic trauma will help us to survive, it is not strange—except perhaps philosophically or theologically—that the human brain, under extended duress, forms such personality compartments. In creating partitioned-off personalities, we divide horrors that would otherwise annihilate us; we can regulate, specialize—and go on living. Viewed in this way, the formation of dissociated ego states is not a disorder, or even an oddity, but rather an adaptation.

The dictionary definition of personality is "the fact or quality of being a person," and by this description, each human being, certainly including Julia, has precisely one personality. But the *psychological definition of personality* is "a relatively enduring set of traits and behavior patterns," and by this definition, a human brain may form many such, should the need arise.

As for naming the "sets"—Tom, Dick, Harry, Amelia, Kate—one of the most dominant features of human psychology is that we are inclined to name absolutely everything, from the instant we are old enough to do so. We name things consciously, as in naming a new baby or a new place. And when we are not consciously aware, we continue to name things, the most apparent examples being the myriad people, places, and objects we name in our dreams, often quite cannily. Dissociated ego states do not always have names; but when they do, their named status is only minimally surprising.

I am sure Julia heard very little of what I had to say during those thirty minutes. I would remember to repeat many times during future sessions, as Julia came to terms with discoveries about her life, and about how her resourceful mind had adapted to her life. She did hear me say that she was not a lunatic, but I greatly doubt she believed me on that particular day.

She noticed the sparkling bracelet in her lap, replaced it onto her wrist, and stared at it miserably. Then she began to touch the violet stones, one by one, with a fingertip of the other hand.

"Some pieces of me broke off from the rest. What do I do now?" she asked me, almost pleadingly.

"Well, at least now you know there's a part of you who's childlike, and a part of you who's tough. The question is—what do you do about the pieces of you now that you know about them?"

"Why didn't I know about them before?"

I answered, "Because consciousness is small."

By this remark, I meant that the self-aware function we refer to as "consciousness" operates in all circumstances as a neurological tool—a mental sentry—admitting and organizing relatively tiny amounts of information from our minds and from the outside world. This mental sentry allows us to function in our day-to-day lives, and not be overwhelmed with input. From moment to moment, "consciousness" does not apprehend the whole of the mind, any more than it apprehends the whole of the world.

To illustrate the limitations of consciousness, a distinguished science writer from Denmark, Tor Nørretranders, has borrowed the term "user illusion" from the field of computer science. The "user illusion" is the way in which the user of a computer conceives of the operations of that computer. At any given moment, a human being, working away, is aware of only the modest amount of information that appears neatly on the computer screen, rather than the almost inconceivable quantities of information used by, or available to, the machine.

Upon even the briefest reflection, most of us understand that the images on the screen, along with whatever rudimentary understanding we may have of what actually goes on in the computer to furnish those images, certainly do not comprise the totality of what is happening inside the box. And yet we energetically resist a conception of our own minds as anything more than the meager contents grudgingly revealed to us by the deftly circumscribed screen of our conscious awareness.

To be ripped suddenly away from the illusion, as Julia had just been, can be painful and frightening. But it is an illusion, and one best left behind.

"Does this mean I have multiple personality disorder?" Julia asked warily.

"No," I said. "Your dissociated ego states probably influence your behavior, which is an extremely important thing to know, but they stay inside your head. We don't have any reason to think they replace you and interact with other people."

"You mean this 'Amelia' and this 'Kate' don't go around talking to my friends?"

"Right."

"Which is to say that some people have dissociated ego states, as you call them, that *do* go around talking to other people?"

"In a sense, yes."

"Oh my God!" Julia moaned theatrically, trying to restore herself with a shade of her usual irony. "How embarrassing!"

Her eyes still frightened, she smiled at me, and I smiled back.

There would be more hard days like this, but Julia was slowly getting better. Raising her memories from underground and making them "regular" was a harrowing process, and involved discoveries that would rock anyone's sense of self to its foundation. But through even this, through her fright—and her embarrassment—Julia's courage had held. I could now be reasonably certain that she would continue to turn on the lights, no matter what.

CHAPTER FIVE

The Human Condition

Neurosis is the way of avoiding non-being by avoiding being.

—Paul Tillich

We are a thoroughly shell-shocked species. Though we have not all suffered abuse as children, we have all endured experiences that we perceived as terrifying, and that utterly exhausted our tender attempts to comprehend and cope. From a troubled world that often seems to menace, many of us have absorbed repeated, toxic doses of secondary trauma as well, from people we care about, and even from an impersonal media. And as a result of our histories, and of our inborn disposition to become dissociative when our minds need protection, moderately dissociated awareness is the *normal mental status* of all adult human beings. Our condition undiscovered, we all behave a little like my trauma patient Julia.

Dissociative behavior is not always tragic, by any means. Often it is benign, and depending upon what is at stake in the moment, it may even be mildly comical.

Consider Matthew of the dish-demolishing mother, twenty-six years later, at age thirty-five. He has grown into an attractive, likable fellow. He lives with his wife in their rural Victorian house, and commutes from there to an enviable professional position in the city. If asked about his childhood, he will offer his sincere opinion that it was basically okay, except for the fact that his parents fought a lot. He will think to himself, and may say aloud, that his own marriage is very different, and he intends to keep it that way. If asked about having children of his own, he will reply that he does not want any. He does not consider himself to be "good father material."

Grown-up Matthew has a sense of humor, and usually enjoys the joke even when it is directed at him. One of the things he gets kidded about the most is a trait his friends call "Matthew's space-cadet routine." From time to time, for no apparent reason, Matthew will simply phase out of the conversation. He and his friends will be discussing something, when all of a sudden Matthew will stop talking—and stop listening—and appear to be lost in some consuming private thought.

"Hey, Matt," someone will say. "What's up?"

When he gets like that, Matthew never responds. He appears to be unaware of the people around him, the very people with whom he was just conversing. His eyes are open, but he does not seem to be looking at anything in particular.

His friends always laugh at him.

"Earth to Matthew. Earth to Matthew," someone will say. But he does not come out of it until one of them playfully punches him in the shoulder, or swats him on the head with a newspaper.

"Where'd you go that time, Matt?"

He always says that he does not know, and invariably, he has forgotten what they were all talking about before. When they tell him that he was doing his space-cadet routine again, he laughs with them, sheepishly. The teasing is almost always in fun.

Less amusing are the discussions he sometimes has with his wife concerning his space-cadet tendencies. She does not use the same cute name for his behavior, instead referring to it as "Matthew's coward thing." Matthew and his wife do not argue often, but when they do, his wife is consistently frustrated by the fact that Matthew tunes out whenever the conversation gets the least bit heated. She complains in the following sort of way: "I can't show even the tiniest bit of anger or emotion around him. When I do, he just turns off, like a computer going down. The eyes go blank. He won't speak. I might as well not be in the room. And the more upset I get, the more he just tunes out. He looks like a zombie. I'm sick of it. I just can't be emotionless all the time."

Matthew's wife is not at all the rageful, scary person his mother was; and yet, even a temperate show of emotion on her part triggers a dissociative episode in Matthew. As for his "space-cadet routine" in other situations, the triggers are not apprehended by his friends, nor even by Matthew. Most often, the triggers are conversational topics that he unconsciously connects, sometimes in quite roundabout ways, with uncomfortable feelings or life pressures. For example, a trivial remark about a colleague's car might spark a free association in Matthew's mind to the fact that he cannot really afford the new Mercedes he would like to have, which thought arouses a strong, irrational feeling of not having enough control over his life. Or a casual comment about the proposed construction of a hospital complex down the street might act as an unnerving reminder that his father, who lives far away, has been ill lately. Similar subjective juxtapositions occur in all people, and in Matthew they trigger a dissociative reaction so instantaneously that he does not have the chance to make a conscious evaluation of his own thoughts and feelings.

He blanks out. His friends do not know why. Eventually, they punch him, and he comes back to himself. He has no memory of his mental absence, nor of the feelings that triggered it, nor of the conversation that came previously. He is just a space cadet. To muddle matters still more, a subject that triggers him on one occasion may not do so at another time, if he happens to be less tired or less anxious generally, or is simply thinking about something else.

Matthew's friends marvel that he can be so successful and smart, and so out to lunch at the same time. They figure he must have some kind of absentminded professor syndrome.

They are ignorant of the fact, and so is Matthew himself, that Matthew's childhood was spent in an atmosphere of trauma that taught him, and then over-taught him, a dissociative strategy of mind. Whenever events got overwhelming in his parents' home, he departed from himself. And over the years, this strategy developed into a mental muscle exercised so often that, now, it is always first to act when Matthew is threatened—by anything—no matter how nontraumatic or insubstantial. As an adult, he does not require his parents' out-of-control spectacles, or any other traumatic stressor, to initiate his dissociative behavior; a moderately uncomfortable thought may do the trick, or a slightly emotional exchange with his wife, or sometimes just being cut off in traffic. Most remarkably, another person's expressed emotion may trigger Matthew even when the feeling is a positive one, such as excited anticipation, passion, or sympathetic concern.

Matthew's dissociative episodes are brief, typically lasting a few minutes, or at most an hour or two. The two-hour events are usually reserved for emotional discussions with his wife. His dissociative behavior is invisible to him, so that when he is alone afterward, he is never cognizant of having departed from himself. In truth, an uninvolved observer would note that, overall, Matthew's dissociative reactions influence Matthew himself far less than they affect the people around him.

How do the dissociative tendencies of someone like Matthew differ from those of Julia, who survived such extreme abuse?

For the most part, there are differences in degree only. If we elaborate upon the "space cadet" image, we can say that, when he is triggered, Matthew gets shot to the moon, but Julia, having been more profoundly traumatized, sometimes gets blasted all the way into deep space. Her episodes last longer, sometimes for days, and for the duration of them, she is irretrievable; she cannot be brought back to herself by a friendly thump on the head, as Matthew can be (except during arguments with his wife).

Across individuals, these variations in degree are related to how much of the mind has been enlisted to cope with traumatic experience. This is determined by the age of the person when the trauma occurred (younger being worse, for neurological as well as psychological reasons), how many times it happened, and its severity. The severity of a trauma is measured by how damaging it was, of course, but also, as we have seen in the previous chapter, by the subjective meaning the victim attaches to it. In this regard, because we all depend so inescapably upon other people, traumas perpetrated by human beings may well require more extensive cognitive acrobatics than do natural or accidental disasters. Moreover, for the same dependency reasons, the actions of a family member may constitute a more severe trauma than the same abuse inflicted by a stranger.

The terrifying occurrences in Julia's childhood were more frequent, more intentional, and in some sense "worse" than the traumas in Matthew's past. Her cognitive apparatus grew even more extensively devoted to trauma-survival than did his. Her dissociative episodes are therefore lengthier and more tenacious. But aside from these differences in extent of dissociative reaction—and whether or not the individuals are in therapy—Julia and Matthew are alike. As an adult, Julia ended up with almost no memory of the specific traumatic events in her life. So did Matthew. After she has been triggered, Julia can still shop for amethyst jewelry, and perform other complex activities. This phenomenon is precisely the same one that allows Matthew to continue driving his car after he has been triggered.

The fact that Julia is in therapy—and Matthew, in the foregoing, is not—bears some elaboration, because this distinction, along with its potential results, is truly the most important one. People, even those like Julia, almost never seek therapy on account of their dissociative behavior alone, which is sometimes invisible to them. They enter therapy for other reasons, for problems that are not only apparent, but also tremendously disruptive: major depression, complete social rejection, suicide attempts, intractable eating disorders, panic attacks, chronic nightmares, addictions, and so forth. In other words, people seek treatment only when they are in substantial pain, and usually only when they have been in pain for a very long time. If dissociative inclinations had been all that Julia suffered from, I might never have met her. Julia came to therapy because she was agonized by depression, and with mounting urgency was knocking on death's door.

Astonishingly, this kind of pain can sometimes hold the kernel of an advantage, for those with sufficient courage to search. Because she was forced by her misery to get help, Julia has identified her dissociative disorder, and has the chance to do something about it. For her suffering, she may in the long run be equipped to take real responsibility for her actions, to conduct her own life in the fullest sense.

Matthew, in contrast, will probably never suffer anything one might legitimately call psychological agony. Instead, he will increasingly accept an absentminded professor identity, and wear it like a coat. If he is introspective, he may wonder, in a detached sort of way, how his general intellect can be so intact while his memory is sometimes so poor. He will come to think of his wife as much too emotionally demanding, and will no doubt tell her so, again and again. He will be scared to have children, and eventually his marriage may (or may not) fall apart. If his marriage does end, the divorce will feel like the worst thing that has ever happened to him, and he will never understand that the loss was largely his responsibility. In short, following from his moderately (but not profoundly) traumatic childhood, neither hapless Matthew's personal identity, nor his own life, will ever be entirely his.

Emotional agony is like physical pain, in that it is a danger signal, forcing us to notice that something is wrong, and to respond. Should a person with a fractured leg feel insufficient pain, he might continue to use his leg, and come to die of gangrene, a swift and pernicious decay.

But here is what might bring someone like Matthew to the changes he needs to make, though he will never be motivated by unbearable anguish: let us say that Matthew's character structure happens to include an abiding sense of personal responsibility for his own behavior, especially for the impact of that behavior on other people. This characteristic of Matthew's would, among its many other worthy effects, render him unable to view his wife as the predominant cause of their difficulties. He would—and the importance of this simple circumstance cannot be overstated—wonder what he was doing to generate unhappiness. *He would wonder whether there might be some way he could change.* And this one honest thought, this single reaction, could make all the difference in the world for someone like Matthew.

With such a character structure, he would be less likely to see his wife as too emotionally demanding, and might wonder what was preventing him from meeting more of her needs. In fact he would be able to see her more clearly in general, because by his nature he would be disinclined to project blame upon her (or upon anyone else). She, for her part, would be far less likely to see him as a "coward," because he would not be one. By most definitions, this Matthew would be rather a brave soul.

And when his wife, and all of his friends, insisted that he was doing something disruptive on a regular basis—spacing out—he still would not understand, but he would not dismiss it. He would, by virtue of his character, feel accountable for his behavior, and for this curious thing that everyone was reporting. He would come to see that he was causing distress, especially to his wife, and for this reason, he would feel distress, too, the more so because he would not automatically know how to remedy the situation.

Other issues also, rationalized and then ignored by an irresponsible person, would be taken into serious account by a responsible Matthew. He would wonder *why.* For example, he would wonder why he could not bear the thought of having children. And should his wife start talking divorce, he would almost inevitably see this as a personal failure, and begin to search, perhaps desperately, for a way to stop the clock on his ticking bomb. And if he were very dedicated, he might well succeed.

Matthew might even reach the point of entering therapy, though he fears this as something that carries an instant label of "crazy person," at least in his opinion. Once in therapy, Matthew would begin to feel scary things, feelings, sensations, and images that had for years been hidden away in the dissociated closets of his mind. In the beginning, he would not know what to make of them. He would be confused and frightened—much more confused and frightened than before he began, when all this was safely tucked away—and he might start to think that he really was crazy. Almost certainly, he would think about quitting. After all, therapy is supposed to make a person feel better, and he would not be feeling better; he would be feeling much worse, at least at first.

Then something might happen, maybe not an earth-rattling insight, but something. As before, Matthew's wife might become upset, maybe a little angry over a minor infraction, and she might tell him that they have to talk. Always in the past, "We have to talk," all by itself, caused Matthew to become dissociative, to phase out, before he had even learned what was wrong.

But this time, *this* time, instead of dissociating, he has a memory: His wife says, "We have to talk."

He looks away, and is silent (as usual). She drops into a chair and starts to cry; this is just too much, and it never seems to change. But then, breaking with all precedent, Matthew suddenly speaks.

"You maggot!" he says.

More astonished than insulted, his wife wipes her eyes and says, "Excuse me?"

Pale, a look of surprise on his face, he turns to her and repeats the epithet: "You maggot! You maggot! When Mom got mad at my father, that's what she used to call him. She called him a maggot."

Let us say this Matthew's wife is gentle and astute, and recognizes that, for now anyway, this new development takes precedence over whatever infraction she had begun to address. She says, "God, that's awful. Did you hear her talking like that when you were little?"

"Well, yeah, all the time," he replies, uncertain as to why she would consider this fact about his childhood to be so startling. "They fought all the time. I thought you knew that."

"I did know that. I mean, you've always said they fought a lot, but you never told me she was so vicious."

"You'd say that was vicious?"

"To call your husband a maggot? Right in front of your own little boy? You *wouldn't* call that vicious?"

"No. Well, I mean I guess I never really thought about it. That's just kind of how things were."

"Well, it was vicious, Matt."

In the course of time, Matthew might have more memories, and just as importantly, he might begin to relabel them. With the help of his wife, his therapist, and maybe some of his friends, he might gradually begin to see that his parents' behavior traumatized him when he was a child, that he witnessed some "vicious" exchanges, in which violence, though not put into action, was strongly implied, and genuinely terrifying to the small person stuck in the middle.

And as Matthew remembered the past, and relabeled his memories, the trigger on his dissociative reactions would become less and less sensitive. He would pass through an uncomfortable period of sadness and regret, and considerable anger, but if he stuck it out to the other end, he would no longer be the absentminded professor. He would be Matthew, living his life in the present. He would have himself back. He would have a fair shot at saving his marriage. Someday he might even become a father, a good one, because he could be *present*, to himself, to his wife, and to his children.

Even at this, Matthew might never specifically recall the plate-smashing extravaganza in his mother's kitchen, when he was nine.

Remembering everything, remembering any particular event, would not be necessary. He would have to recall only enough to make the themes of his childhood, the tenor of his past experiences, clear to him. For some people, a single visual image or a powerful phrase or a word ("Maggot!") may be enough of a keyhole into the past to initiate the conscious relabeling and detoxification of a long succession of related traumatic events, not all of which are remembered specifically.

The idea is not to produce a detailed feature film of one's personal history, but rather to allow the brain to recognize some of what happened in the past, and to label it properly—though this may at first be frightening and painful—such that the mind no longer hides from the present as if the foggy, wordless, dissociated past were still ongoing.

The goal, put simply, is to enable oneself to live substantially in the present. The task is life-affirming, and also a kind and generous thing to do for the people one loves.

Achieving this deceptively simple-sounding goal requires work, courage, and a commitment to personal responsibility for one's own life, requires these most especially when the venture has not been motivated by a conspicuous psychiatric disorder. Though his history is perhaps not so colossal as Julia's, this Matthew, the one who takes on his family's dissociative legacy and wins, the one who comes to decide that the buck will stop with him, is someone I would be delighted to know. This Matthew is a person of whom I would be very proud.

Not everyone's dissociative style causes him to be a space cadet like Matthew, at least not all the time. What does dissociative behavior look like in other ordinary people? What does it *feel* like?

There are many dissociative experiences that are not trauma-related, and they feel familiar to most people. A moviegoer sits down to watch *The Fugitive*, and departs from himself for a while, via a highly entertaining trance. Many of us occasionally drive our cars in a trance, not necessarily because we have been triggered, like Matthew, by our own anger at another driver, but for the simple reason that we are alone, and are allowing ourselves to go "somewhere else" mentally. This variety of trance, the daydream that takes one away, is perhaps the most recognizable example of trauma-unrelated mildly dissociative behavior.

Better than neutral, some dissociative tendencies are productive, sometimes magnificently so. Countless talented individuals, among them James Joyce and Albert Einstein, have referred to their need to depart from reality when they were deeply involved in the process of artistic or scientific creation. And most people can recall days when they were so immersed in interesting work that they "lost track of time." These episodes of mental departure can be almost magically fruitful. They do not necessarily involve the partitioning off of trauma, but rather the dissociative leaving behind of normal, everyday "reality" (the clock, other people, most of one's surroundings, hunger, fatigue, and other practical daily concerns), in order to realize a creative endeavor. We may have to deal with other people's annoyance at us when we fall into such trances, especially if we are gifted at them, but in our dissociative getaways that serve the creative process, we are not specifically dealing with trauma.

We are able to identify such experiences. We know how they *feel*. In contrast, dissociative events that have their origins in trauma are more difficult for us to recognize. Trauma-engendered dissociative reactions exist to keep portions of our experience from us, such that we are not paralyzed by our experience, and so by their very nature, the reactions themselves tend to be hidden from us, too. Or to be more exact, they tend to be slippery, hard to grasp, like rivulets of mercury, or dreams after the dreamer has wakened. Most of us have no idea how traumatic dissociation *feels*, until or unless we have an awfully good reason to focus on the project of learning.

As an initial glimpse, I can offer the "near-miss reaction," which will feel familiar to some: in the course of events, sometimes catastrophes almost, but not quite, happen, and we are triggered into dissociation by the *nearly*. For example—it is late afternoon, and you are driving your car due west, into the sun. The glare is blinding, so that you squint even through your sunglasses. You stop at a light, and prepare to make a left turn. Your turn signal is on. The light turns green, you pull left into the intersection, and in the microsecond after your eyes are relieved from the sun's glare, you realize that a cyclist has pulled out directly in front of you, and is barely skirting the front of your moving car on the driver's side. For one heartbeat, you see the cyclist's face, which is alarmed and indignant. You have avoided each other, and there is no accident; but if you had set off just a little bit faster . . .

You brake, and remain in the intersection for a moment before continuing. You can feel your blood pressure rise up to your ears, and you curse the cyclist for what you are sure was his recklessness. You figure the rest of your afternoon is ruined, because you are so upset and angry.

But by the time you are half a mile away, the incident has left your mind, and you are thinking about something else. Another mile, and the whole thing might as well not have happened, except—that night, at three in the morning, you wake in the safety of your bed and, for an instant, you see the cyclist in your mind, as if he were a snapshot. Suddenly, you remember that you almost had a serious accident earlier. Your heart races, and then slows again. You realize that you had totally forgotten about the incident until just now. For a moment, you have the sense that time has somehow collapsed: you were in that intersection looking at the scornful cyclist's face, and now—presto—you are here in your bed.

You forgot the occurrence not because it was technically traumatic (it was not), but because it was alarming, and being ambushed in this way tripped the wire on dissociative proclivities established long before you were old enough to have the car keys.

Countless other circumstances trip the same wire. Another trigger that may be recognizable to some is performance anxiety, which is what we sometimes feel when we must accomplish a task of personal significance before an audience of one or more other people. Common examples of performance anxiety are giving a speech, appearing on camera, being called on in a class, having a part in a play or a recital, hosting an event, or simply walking into a room populated with people we consider attractive or important. All of these situations, though not traumatic, may generate enough anxiety to set off our preestablished dissociative reactions.

Consider a bride at her wedding. She and her groom have been planning this day for months. Now, she is scared out of her wits, not so much to get married, she tells herself, but rather to go through with the elaborately anticipated performance of the wedding itself. She dresses in an outrageous white dress that she has obsessed about for as long as she can remember, and takes her beaming father's arm. The first phrases of the relevant tune issue forth from the organ, and clutching her father, she begins to travel a path through all the people who are important, or ever have been important, in her life. Faces swim around her. Now she is genuinely not certain that she will be able to walk the required distance. She can no longer feel her feet as they move her forward. For that matter, she can scarcely feel anything. She has a sense of being out of body, an impression that she is floating a little above herself, and that her body is now acting on its own.

When she gets to the front of the room, and her husband-to-be is standing there, she finds that she can still recite the words they rehearsed, but she has absolutely no idea how loud her voice is. Maybe she is whispering inaudibly, or maybe she is fairly shouting; she simply cannot discern. Far from feeling warm and close to her husband, she is quite unable even to get back into herself. But she gets through the vows, and no one but her notices anything unusual about her mental status.

At the wedding reception, the bride is lighter than air. She laughs and talks with everyone, she drinks champagne, she dances, she cuts the cake. But sometime after it is all over, she will realize that there is a four-hour gap in her memory. She has mental snapshots from the party after the ceremony, a face here, a sentence there, a sense of activity and celebration; but overall, she cannot remember her own wedding, nor most of the wedding reception. Two weeks later, when she views the videotape, she will be amazed to see how entirely composed she looked and sounded during those same four hours.

As with our depersonalized bride, a nonclinical dissociative episode can feel like an out-of-body event and a partial failure of memory; or as with the "near-miss reaction," it can feel like a brief collapse of time; or as with Matthew, it can feel like nothing at all, until or unless some other person gets amused or frustrated.

Yet another common type of dissociative reaction is usually referred to as *flashback*. In literature and film, a flashback is often simply the portrayal of a memory. A psychological flashback is more profound; it is *being there* once more, living through a past event, or some part of it, again in one's mind. As such, a flashback involves dissociating from present reality and jumping back in time to re-experience past events, often just for a moment or two, but in severe cases, for hours or even days. The woman reading a newspaper at the depot, Beverly, who momentarily "smelled" nonexistent chlorine when she was jolted by the train's whistle, was having a short-lived flashback.

Lengthy, unremitting flashbacks are an extremely difficult clinical issue, heartbreaking to witness, even for a seasoned clinician. They are the result of profound and chronic trauma, and can be unspeakably painful. In striking contrast with the gamut of other dissociative reactions, flashbacks do not provide an escape from fear, but rather an hallucinatory return to hideous images and feelings from a traumatized past. The person who experiences repeated, lengthy flashbacks is consigned to a torment that cannot be compared with anything in our ordinary lives. Hounded by the past, she may end up in a tight fetal curl on the floor, irretrievably lost in her own hell for hours at a time.

Brief flashbacks, however, are not uncommon, and most of us have had one at some time or other, most typically when we were very tired, sleep-deprived, or physically ill.

As an illustration, early in the years of my practice, during and after a visit to the nation of Haiti, I gained some unbidden experience of my own with the haunting outcomes of even brief traumatic exposure. In fact, traveling outside of our buffered "first" world, I have often been brought eye-to-eye with the faces of hardship and trauma, and the effects of these upon the mind.

From that trip, the spot I remember most vividly—and the place that most eludes whatever power of mind I have—is a bedroom, specifically the bedroom of the Sir John Gielgud Suite of the Grand Hotel Oloffson, in Port-au-Prince. Before it was destroyed in the 1986 uprising that sent the incumbent despot Baby Doc Duvalier copiously packing to France, the Grand Hotel Oloffson existed as an ornate and genuine Victorian mansion, set on a hillside that elevated it somewhat above the busy, dignified despair of the city. The hotel appeared to the eye as white nineteenth-century spires in constant danger of being smothered by tropical vegetation. And on the inside, this implausible castle was as beautiful as a child's fantasy.

The bedroom—where, in my mind's eye, I can even now see myself standing—is wicker, white linen, lace, and Haitian wall paintings, a mixture of powdered Victorian style and bursting Haitian energy. There is a high four-poster bed made up in white linen and white lace pillow covers, a large dresser with a beveled mirror, and dominating the room, a massive floor-to-ceiling wardrobe with ornate double doors. All is whitewashed, every wall, every article of furniture. And over the whitewash, every available surface is lavished with Haitian art, here an original painting in a lacquered wooden frame, there a hand-painted mural embellished with inscrutable and yet oddly familiar images.

West Indian sunlight enters through tall Victorian windows, and plays with the edges of shadows that slow-waltz around the room, and then melt away. A wind, hot but not deadly, billows floor-length white linen curtains into ceaseless movement, and seems to inspirit other things as well, sashes, my clothing, doors. My baggage is by the swaying door to a breezy hotel corridor. All is in languid motion, except for me. I am standing quite still between the enigmatically painted wardrobe and the bed.

The scene is mesmerizing, like a dream of permanent summer. Coming from somewhere outside the great windows is the muffled sound of someone playing steel drums. Perhaps this person is rehearsing a piece, because musical phrases stop in the middle, are repeated, stop again. Like wind chimes, I think to myself.

I remember the Sir John Gielgud Suite far better than I remember the voodoo ceremony I witnessed that night, because my memory of the latter is clouded by fear. I do recall that the grizzled driver of the antique Ford seemed to be laughing at us as he drove me and my companion to the ritual, and laughing even more knowingly afterward, as he took us back to the hotel. He had been offered ten American dollars for the job—two weeks' wages at least, in Haiti—and I had bargained only for an interesting experience, an underestimation I should not have made.

Haiti is one of the poorest nations on earth, and as we left Port-au-Prince for the countryside, the outskirts of the city moved past the taxi windows in a panorama of poverty and deprivation too savage to be completely taken in at first. The roadway was lined with what Americans would perceive as lean-to sheds and large cardboard boxes arranged sideways, shed after box after shed—what those who lived here thought of as their houses. The late Haitian dusk had finally arrived, but there remained enough light to make out a landscape, barely seven hundred miles from Florida, that most of us would experience as a nightmare (for we would be able to relate to it only as a dream), a phantasm of danger, smothering grime, and despair.

I could see into the cardboard "houses" well enough to catch the indecipherable staccato movements of large and small human shadows, and an occasional illuminated face. From time to time, someone standing by the road would wave at the driver, calling out his name, and he would wave back.

"I'm famous," he explained in careful English. "I have a car."

Of all this, the most lasting image for me is the just-perceptible face of a painfully gaunt little boy, about six years old I would guess, who poked his head out of a dwelling like a young turtle, and grinned at us as we passed. His guileless smile was full of missing teeth, like any six-year-old's would be.

The ceremony to which I was escorted took place outdoors, at a special meeting place in the woods. By the time we were seated underneath the ancient banyan tree that was the consecrated temple, the night had come. We saw by moonlight and by torchlight. I do not know how long I was there, and my fear has left me with only a few hazy mental pictures. I remember that there was steady, hypnotic drumming, chanting. There was a priest, and a priestess dressed in virginal white lace, and dancing, screaming, the implied threat of violence, violation, perhaps even death. A chicken was sacrificed, and the blood from its gushing neck was splattered everywhere, particularly upon the white vestments of the priestess. The drumming became louder, numbing. Coals were spread over the ground, and set ablaze until they glowed red, and a miasma of bitter smoke devoured what had been the last comfort, the soothing smells of trees and earth.

A man, not the priest, another man, began to walk on the fire, the skin of his bare feet directly upon the superheated coals. But this was not gruesome enough. He then reached down with his hand, picked up a red coal, and popped it into his mouth as if it were a large piece of candy. He bellowed like a wounded animal at first, but then was silent. And to my horror, he next looked over at me as if he had known me all my life, and slowly but purposefully gyrated toward where I was sitting.

I say with great honesty that at that moment I could not have fled or even moved if my life had depended on it, and I was far from sure that it did not.

He approached until his face was only about a foot from mine, stared penetratingly into my eyes, and opened his mouth to reveal the chunk of coal still glowing red-hot on his tongue. While the drums pounded, he continued to stare into me in this way—again, for how long I am not certain—and what I saw in his eyes can be described only as the specter of emptiness. It was as though his soul had left him altogether. I was forced by this man, whether by magic or by artifice is not important, to look directly into the eyes of the void.

After it was all over, the driver reappeared from the shadows, and silently led me out of the trees and back to his car, as if he knew very well, and was secretly amused, that I would not be able to speak for a while. Seldom have I been so glad to see anyone. On the way back to the hotel, I recalled, all in a start, that my suite had no locks on the windows or doors. Warm as the air was, I felt like a column of cold clay instead of flesh. I do not remember how I slept that night, or whether I even went to bed.

However, after I got back to where I now live in Massachusetts—like anyone who has been scared half to death, but then finds herself ensconced again in her usual life—I thought of it as over. Nearly five years later, five years of viewing the experience as only an interesting tale to tell, I learned that it was not over at all.

A hoodlum of a virus had confined me to my bed, with a fever just short of delirium. It was January in New England, and winds from a baby nor'easter sopped and huffed at the windows around me. I pulled the blankets up closer to my nose, and longed for the oblivion of sleep. But whenever I fell asleep, I had the same frightening hypnagogic vision, the same flashback. Each time slumber began to envelop my consciousness, I dreamt—no, I *believed*—that I was not in my own bed at home, but rather back in that high four-poster bed in the Sir John Gielgud Suite of the Grand Hotel Oloffson.

The white lace pillow covers were there instead of my plain ones, and the cryptic murals, the billowing linen curtains, the open doorways, and of course the great painted wardrobe. But instead of muted music from steel drums, I heard malignant drumming and chanting, exactly as they had sounded under the ceremonial banyan tree, and every bit as loud. The dancers were there. The priestess was there. Or they might as well have been, where my personal reality was concerned. Most alarming, I could not see them. They were hiding from me.

If I did not manage to wrest myself from sleep at this point in the dream—which I did do, over and over again—the vision would then continue to its next chapter, in which the heavy double doors of the Victorian wardrobe would swing slowly open, and the man with the soulless eyes, the coal-walker, would be revealed standing inside. Dressed in a long white tunic, he had no coals, but instead held in his hand a lighted white candle. He floated out of the cabinet toward me, and in my dream, I would marvel that the candle continued to burn despite the January wind.

I would always wake just then, shivering violently, in part from the fever, and in part from my terror. And I have no doubt that he is there yet, somewhere inside my brain, just waiting for the mercury to rise.

Under the banyan tree that night, and later in my sickbed at home, I was forced to understand how fear affects the mind—and how easily some people can use hardship and fear to paralyze and control their fellow human beings. (Before his departure, Baby Doc was secretly considered by most Haitians to be the supreme practitioner of voodoo.) Also, I learned something about the alchemistic nature of *memory*, and the way memory can collude with imagination to make our own lives mysterious to us. Sometimes memory is as clear and precise as the sound of a grandmother's singing voice in church, and sometimes as murky as what one actually witnessed in a dark Haitian forest. I was forcefully reminded, as well, that we all live inside our own heads. Experiences, and especially other people, powerfully affect our internal universe, to be sure; but we live deep inside of that universe, always.

·   ·   ·

Leaving flashback, but still chasing the rivulets of common dissociative experience and how it *feels*—let us examine some events in
three other lives, beginning with the experience of demifugue:

Laura, a college sophomore, is on an airplane flying home for
the Thanksgiving break. She has been contentedly studying during
the trip, but as the plane begins to land, she puts away her books
and notices that her stomach has started to hurt, and that she feels
unaccountably tired. She is glad to see that the lights of evening
are twinkling on below; soon, she can crawl into her childhood bed
and go to sleep. Laura's parents meet her at the airport. Her father
is sullen, which is not unusual. Laura thinks he has been drinking
again. She notices that her mother designates herself as the driver
for the ride home. Her father says almost nothing, and her mother,
who can be something of a space shot, chatters over the silence.

When they arrive at her parents' house, Laura proclaims that
her stomach hurts a lot, and that she is going to bed. Closing herself into the comfort of her old room, she sleeps deeply for twelve
hours. But when she finally gets up, she is still so tired that she can
barely keep her eyes open. She tries to help her mother put the fin-
ishing touches on the Thanksgiving meal, but she is dragging; her
slender body feels like it weighs a thousand pounds. When the
guests arrive, Laura is quiet and withdrawn. She feels like a spectator, rather than a participant. And, vaguely, she reflects that there
is much for a spectator to watch; some of her relatives are real
characters, "strong personalities," as her mother would say. When
the gargantuan turkey is placed on the dining table, Laura's grandmother, dressed entirely in pink velour, and already tipsy, stands
and leads everyone (except Laura) in a full-volume performance of
"Over the River and through the Woods to Grandmother's House
We Go."

As the hours pass, Laura feels more and more distant from
everyone, dreamy and silent. She is so sleepy that she feels a bit unreal, detached, almost as if she were watching her family's Thanksgiving gathering through the wrong end of some strange
telescope.

Laura remains irrepressibly sleepy for three more days. On Sunday evening, she wearily boards a flight back to school. She assumes that the return trip will finish her off, and has already decided to skip her Monday morning class. But to her surprise, when the pilot announces that the plane is about to land, Laura feels awake and alert for the first time since Wednesday. When she gets back to her dorm room, she stays up until two, with her friends.

For whatever emotional reasons, and there are probably a number, Laura has been derealized, detached—dissociative—while at her childhood home.

Next, let us follow Kenneth, as he takes his young son on an outing to the top of one of the World Trade towers.

Kenneth is afraid of heights. Moreover, he is ashamed of the fact that he is afraid of heights, and tries to keep his secret, especially from his six-year-old son, Trevor. Trevor is not afraid of heights, and perversely, is possessed of a keen wish to visit the observation deck of the World Trade Center, which one of his friends at school went to, afterward proclaiming it "mega-cool." Kenneth promised to take Trevor there someday, and now it would seem that someday has arrived.

As they go up in the elevator at Two World Trade Center—and up and up and up—Kenneth feels queasy already. When the doors slide open, Trevor sets off in a sprint toward the big windows. Kenneth snags him by the arm, and makes a little prepared speech: "Cool your jets, Trevor. In a crowded place like this, you should walk very slowly. Let's just take our time. We'll get to the glass in a minute or two."

Trevor looks at his father as if he were crazy, but he complies. Finally, they complete their drawn-out approach to the north perimeter of the observatory. Trevor exclaims and asks questions— "What's that water over there, Daddy?"—while Kenneth stands back a few feet and cautiously leans forward from the waist, as if he were peering over a windy cliff. One hundred and seven heart-stopping stories below, Kenneth's beloved Manhattan leers up at him in the form of a sunny, steaming panorama, seemingly infinite, and definitely bottomless. The experience is intolerable for him, and he steps back. He tells Trevor that he will just have a seat over there, while Trevor looks. Fortunately, Trevor is so enchanted by the giant vista that he ignores his father's behavior; but he does look a little downcast when his father adamantly refuses to attend the free motion-simulated helicopter ride through New York City.

By the time they get back down to Liberty Street, Kenneth is feeling strange, not at all himself, as if there had just been some odd paradigm shift in his thinking. Normally optimistic and affable, he now feels distressingly paranoid and alienated. Only Trevor seems to be exempted from Kenneth's sense of estrangement. He clasps his son's arm as they walk along, and keeps as much distance as possible from the hordes of other people, no easy task. Each time a stranger glances at him, or at Trevor, Kenneth feels an inexplicable surge of anger. When someone a few yards away steps into the street at the wrong time and nearly gets hit by a car, Kenneth mutters an obscene insult under his breath. Trevor regards his father quizzically. Kenneth himself wonders where on earth this sudden misanthropy has come from, and feels a little foolish.

But he continues to be suspicious and angry at everything, into the evening at home. He thinks he may have had this peculiar feeling before, once or twice, and knowing he is in the mood to pick a fight, he avoids his wife. He has trouble falling asleep, because he is ruminating about all the things in his life that are making him mad. However, to his relief, when he wakes up in the morning, after a night full of dreams he cannot remember, the paranoia has passed, and he feels like himself. As the morning goes on, he perceives that he is at peace with the world once again.

Kenneth's own childhood was troubled, and yet—bitter to realize—a common enough story all over the world. His Russian immigrant parents named him Kenneth because the name seemed so all-American. When his father's job allowed, they moved to a middle-class neighborhood that was a long commute from the city, and that, unfortunately for the eight-year-old Kenneth, contained no other "foreign" families. Little Kenneth, who was a moderate and people-loving boy, tried valiantly to conceal from his parents the bruises and occasional bloody noses inflicted upon him by the neighborhood bullies, who had been taught indirectly, and sometimes not so indirectly, to hate people who were different. At times, he privately feared that his mother and father might be in danger, too, even though they were big. And of course, he felt that there must be something woefully wrong with him and his whole family.

Before long, little Kenneth slipped into a state of lethargy that mystified and frightened his parents, and made them feel helpless to do anything for him. His depression did not start to lift until he was about fourteen—and nearly six feet tall, no longer a very inviting target for his persecutors. The confrontations ceased, and as he appeared to become "himself" again, smiling and amiable, his parents were filled with relief, and decided between them not to rock the boat by asking too many questions about the dark years that had just passed.

Kenneth's history is an illustration of the ways in which an atmosphere of bigotry, entirely by itself, can overwhelm a small child's sensibilities and his belief in his ability to cope. But today, Kenneth's life is different. In a gradual and natural progression, he has indeed become an all-American, indistinguishable in speech, behavior, and interests, from any other all-American man. He has forgotten his early depression, and most of the worst things that happened to him in the malevolent neighborhood of his childhood, and has established a reasonably contented life back in New York City. Certainly, his son Trevor knows nothing at all of his father's early ordeals. And if you were to ask Kenneth about what it is like to be a newcomer to this country, he would say, in all good humor, that you would have to ask his parents. He really does not know.

But Kenneth's secret fright at one hundred and seven stories above the ground was intense enough to trigger the influence of a protective dissociated ego state, formed long ago for reasons entirely other than heights. Whether or not Kenneth's ego state has a hidden name is unknown, but its attitudes are similar to those of "Kate," my patient Julia's protective, belligerent ego state discovered under hypnosis. Struggling with the influence of a dissociated ego state is a fairly common experience, and one that is nearly always misattributed ("I'm in such a strange mood today," and, "I've got to snap out of this," etc.). When triggered, an old ego state may present itself whole, like a nursery rhyme learned before fluent speech and stored tenaciously in the mind, at primitive and powerful levels.

The difference between being affected by an ego state, like Kenneth or Julia, and switching completely to a dissociative identity, as in dissociative identity disorder (formerly called multiple personality disorder), is that a person merely influenced by a dissociated ego state retains an *observing ego*, which is simply the capacity to observe and evaluate one's self. Kenneth's observing ego (a faculty that he continues to perceive as a part of Kenneth, as an aspect of his true and usual self) realizes that something unusual is happening to Kenneth's internal experience, and takes what measures it can to subvert the alien feelings and thoughts, and to direct Kenneth's behavior in a mainly Kenneth-like fashion. When dissociated ego states are triggered, whether one retains or loses the observing ego is a crucial distinction. It makes the difference between being uncomfortably divided within one's self, like Kenneth, and being utterly replaced for a while by an "alter ego."

We are all without an observing ego sometimes, in fact every time we lose ourselves utterly in a movie or a daydream. This absence of observing ego is a part of why dissociated ego states that actually take over feel "embarrassing" and out of control to most people—in a way similar to our embarrassment when someone catches us in an intense reverie: we know we have not been watching ourselves.

I would try to glorify humankind by saying that, in the observing ego, we have at last found the feature that distinguishes us from the other animals—which for some reason we are obsessed with doing—but that I would not be surprised to find that elephants, certain large birds, the great apes (and maybe even cats and dogs) have observing egos, too. For any of us, primate or human, observing ego is not conscience or transcendent function or consciousness itself or soul. It is simply, and profoundly, the part of us that watches us.

Laura, the student, entered a demifugue state while at her childhood home, though nothing officially traumatic happened there during her Thanksgiving break. She was certainly not familiar with the term "demifugue," but she—and her observing ego—knew that something was very wrong for four days, and that whatever it was lifted when she got back to school. Kenneth, the daddy, evoked an old dissociated ego state while trying to conceal his fear of heights. Still able to observe himself, he wondered where the compelling misanthropy had come from all of a sudden, and he was most relieved when it had passed.

Now, let us spend a few moments with a new grandmother, Cleo, on her return flight from visiting her newborn grandson.

Cleo's whimsical mother, who predicted accurately that this time she would have a black-haired daughter who would be named Cleopatra, died in childbirth. As an infant, Cleo went home to her grief-stricken father and her four older brothers. A concerned and affectionate aunt had moved in for the first two years, to help out; but after that, pretty, black-haired Cleo had more or less fended for herself, in a raucous household dominated by motherless young boys. She was never intentionally abused, but suffered the overpowering and often dangerous circumstances left to small children who must somehow get through the day without maternal supervision or protection. Everyone in her world was larger and stronger than she, and she was acutely aware of being vulnerable.

The struggles with her brothers overwhelmed her, both physically and emotionally. But oddly, her brothers do not remember things that way. Even these days, as men in their seventies, they will sometimes remark proudly about how fearless a little girl was their baby sister. The adult Cleo just smiles and says nothing, because she does not really recall the fearlessness they are talking about, and she has some difficulty picturing herself in wrestling matches with these four gentlemen in the first place.

"No matter how much she got hurt, or got her back against the wall, she never let on her feelings. She put a blank look on her face. It was grand. You should have seen the wee trouper!"

There were a number of solitary times, also, when she got herself into scrapes that, but for a bit of Irish luck, might well have meant her life. When she was five, for example, she climbed up to the roof of the house, as she had seen some older children do, and slipped off a beam, landing flat on her back on the dry earth. The fall left her unable to move or inhale for several moments, during which she thought she might die. When finally she could breathe again, she picked herself up without calling for help, and went to her room. She sat on the edge of the bed for a while, and allowed her feelings to recede from her automatically, like a loud noise that, simply by the laws of physics, dissipates to silence in the far distance. When she got up from the bed, she was calm.

Despite its near misses, childhood passed, and she survived. Adulthood came, and with it a measure of safety, a good marriage, a full life, and a mistiness regarding certain realities of the long-ago past.

Silver-haired Cleo is now sixty-six years old, and has three grown children of her own. But this is her first grandchild. She feels that she has been waiting forever, since her children grew up, to hold another newborn baby in her arms. When her son called to say that his wife was pregnant, Cleo was ecstatic. After she hung up the phone, she jumped up and down in the middle of the bedroom floor, shouting, "I'm gonna be a grandma! I'm gonna be a grandma!" Her husband laughed at her, but she could tell that, in his own way, he was just as thrilled.

During the next seven months, she spent many afternoons blissfully choosing an extravagant layette. But when the word finally came that labor was in progress, and as she and her husband drove to the airport to catch the next plane from Cincinnati to Chicago,

Cleo was consumed by less comfortable feelings. What if something terrible happened to his son's wife during the birth? What if there were something wrong with the baby? What if they expected her to know all about how to care for a newborn, and she had forgotten? What if her daughter-in-law would not let her spend the amount of time with the baby that she wanted to? What if the other grandma, the *mother's* mother, resented all the baby things she had chosen and already shipped to Illinois? What if she were not really ready to be a grandmother after all? This last question plagued her the most, as the plane made its landing at O'Hare.

But now Cleo is on the plane back to Cincinnati, after a week's visit with the new parents and their perfect newborn son. Everything went fine. All of her worries seem distant, and she feels extremely happy. Seated next to her and her husband, on the aisle, is a nice young woman, more or less her daughter-in-law's age. The young woman converses with Cleo about her trip, and sweetly encourages her to talk about her grandson. Cleo willingly shares some of the adorable things about the baby, such as his virtue of having the world's tiniest feet, and she regrets that her photos are not developed yet.

Finally the woman says, "It must have been so amazing to hold the baby in your arms for the first time. What were you feeling?"

"Yes. Oh yes," replies Cleo. And then she stops. All of a sudden, she realizes (her observing ego "realizes") the strangest thing. As far as she can recall, at that once-in-a-lifetime moment when she had picked up her newborn grandson and held him in her arms for the first time, she had felt absolutely nothing at all—not love, not tenderness, not anxiety, not curiosity—not anything. As a matter of fact, that entire first day is shamefully emotionless in her memory. She can picture what happened, in as much detail as she remembers anything, but she can recall no feelings. The day had occurred, but it had gone by numbly, in unaffecting black-and-white scenes. After all the years of waiting, when she had finally met her first grandchild, there had been no colors, just events.

Cleo's collection of difficult feelings and worries about the birth of her grandchild set off a reaction that temporarily separated her from her own emotions. She would have been competent to manage her various emotions on this nontraumatic occasion if she could have kept them, but she did not have that choice. Her dissociative mental habits, formed by ancient traumas—lonely childhood misadventures, and wrestling matches with grade-school boys—were too entrenched to let her try. Her experience is a good illustration of the way in which our dissociative capacity, evolved to parcel our experience and thus help us to survive, too easily develops into a reflexive grasping arm that can rob a person of important bits and pieces of the very life it has preserved.

Dissociation can be compared to a drug (another human tool that can help or do harm). The ability to dissociate is like having an unlimited supply of a medium-to-good narcotic that never habituates. And by the time we are adults, this mental analgesia is so trigger-happy that trauma or overwhelming fear or pain is no longer required to infuse it; because circumstances are frequently anxiety-provoking or difficult or confusing or just uncertain, we take small potentiated escapes from our present moments. As if even the most sober among us were lifelong addicts, our awareness goes in and out, in and out, often unnoticed, while our overlearned adult behaviors continue apace. Our lives have been this way for such a long time that we do not normally ponder these mental events any more than we normally ponder our own breathing.

The result is that adult human memory performs something like the old-fashioned kinetoscope, a peephole looking onto a winding roll of separate pictures that together simulate a moving, undivided whole. Though we are largely oblivious of the fact, our lives as they advance are lined with countless unwanted blank seams of nonawareness.

Cleo is a loving person, and in the years that follow the birth of her grandson, she proves to be a wonderful grandmother, with all kinds of deeply experienced feelings for the little boy and his parents. But she never forgets, and never tells anyone, that on the day when she met her first grandchild, she simply felt nothing at all.

PART THREE

SPLIT IDENTITY

CHAPTER SIX

Replaced

*Everything can be taken from a man but one thing: the
last of the human freedoms—to choose one's attitude in
any given set of circumstances, to choose one's own way.*

—Viktor Frankl

The first time I encountered someone with floridly apparent
dissociative identity disorder was during my internship at
McLean Hospital. Founded in 1811, in the quiet, affluent
town of Belmont, Massachusetts, just west of Cambridge, McLean
is Harvard Medical School's major psychiatric teaching hospital, a
venerable institution uneasy with its fame as it makes appearances
in novels, autobiographies, film, and even popular song. Much of
the physical facility consists of a collection of mansions, each of
which was built in the nineteenth century to accommodate a single
individual from a wealthy family—not quite "right" enough to remain decorously at home—along with his or her servants. These
tremendous, ivy-smothered houses, long ago divided into multiple
offices and wards to house the many, rest at unobtrusive angles to

narrow roads that wind through acres of dignified old trees, placid lawns, and hilly apple orchards.

Driving through the grounds, one might easily imagine that this is the campus of a fine old New England college, at a time when school is evidently not in session, for very few people are to be seen out of doors, even on a clear, warm afternoon. But then one sees, perhaps, a solitary individual walking along one of the roads, slumped, head down in almost palpable depression, and one's sense of the place begins to shift to something darker.

A substantial contingent of the patient population is still well-to-do and educated, and at any given time may include the world-famous, or the children of the famous, clientele whose identities are meticulously guarded from the curious outside world. The aura of the place, and the privileged, educated status of some of its patients, is permanently represented in my mind by the cosmopolitan graffiti that one of the young residents of the hospital's renowned children's unit once escaped long enough to inscribe in large letters, as if to signal for help, upon an outside wall:

"*LES ADULTES SONT FOUX.*" (The adults are crazy.)

When I was an intern at McLean, outsiders often found the patients indistinguishable from the staff, none of whom wore uniforms; and much to the institution's credit, the VIP inmates were usually indistinguishable from the other patients.

On this particular occasion, I was supervising a community meeting on one of the adult wards, convened each week to address the day-to-day living issues of the dozen or so patients living there at the time. The patients, one psychiatric nurse, one mental health worker, and I sat in an old country kitchen on the ground floor of one of the reappropriated mansions, around an extremely long distressed wood table. A motley assortment of pots and pans and other cookware, conspicuously devoid of knives, hung from hooks on the walls, and a chubby antique refrigerator chugged away in a corner. The windows were dressed in ruffled checkered curtains. In our absence—for we all looked very solemn—the room would likely have been a picture of cheerful country-house domesticity.

The rest of the ward consisted of an entry parlor, a tastefully appointed living room, and six dorm-style double-to-triple bedrooms, three for the women, three for the men. No one, no matter how financially capable, could reserve a private bedroom.

The meeting in the big kitchen began typically enough. There were the usual reticent complaints, and also the customary accusations. One of the men was paying far too much attention to one of the women, and vice versa. (Apart from prison, a psychiatric hospital is the only place in our society where all of an adult's rights may be legally taken away, including, most definitely, freedom of association.) Dishes were being left in the sink unwashed. This one was hogging the telephone. That one was snoring all night.

But then an angry middle-aged woman turned to a younger woman named Crystal, a gentle, retiring person well liked by all the patients and the staff, and waved a finger at her startled, pretty face.

"And *you* are really a jerk!" growled the older woman. "You ate all my Bosc pears!" The hostile woman's blotched skin made her look fierce, and the bulging vessels of her scalp were clearly visible beneath her thinning, almost nonexistent hair.

"I haven't eaten any pears, Fran," Crystal replied softly. And to everyone's chagrin, her dark eyes filled with tears.

"Jesus, Fran. She hardly even eats at all. Shut up, why don't you?" said a third woman.

I *knew*, I had of course been *informed*, that twenty-five-year-old Crystal's diagnosis included violently self-injurious behaviors ("cutting," for example), and also "multiple personality disorder" (the old-fashioned conception for dissociative identity disorder), but my intellectual understanding did nothing to prepare me psychologically for what happened next. It was not that Crystal suddenly looked different—she did not. It was that someone else's voice, altogether someone else's, came out of her mouth.

"I'm scared. I want to go to my room," said the voice, unquestionably that of a three- or four-year-old girl. This voice was so unlike Crystal's own that it seemed disembodied to me, as if it might be playing electronically from some device inside her throat. I was so jolted that I stopped breathing for a moment.

"I'm scared, Dr. Stout. Can I go?" the voice insisted.

I collected myself enough to ask a vaguely appropriate question, "Why are you scared, Crystal?"

One of the other patients, a sad-eyed young man of about Crystal's age, looked at me and, trying hard not to sound insubordinate, corrected my mistake, "It's not Crystal. It's Casey."

"Why are you scared, Casey?" I tried to recoup.

"Fran hates me. She *hates* me," said the otherworldly little voice.

And then "Casey" began to cry in earnest, the authentic, wailing, little-gasp distress sobs of a tiny child, the ones that elicit a knee-jerk protective response from nearly everyone who hears them. All of the patients, even Fran, oriented toward her, stretched out their arms across the long table, tried to take care of her. After a while, she stopped crying, and became disturbingly silent.

When the meeting was over, I immediately went to the nurses' station and wrote an order for Crystal/"Casey" to be placed on "house restriction and thirty-minute checks," meaning that she would not be allowed to leave the ward, and that every half hour, without fail, a staff member with a clipboard would locate her, and note her whereabouts on a form. These safety checks (safety from herself) would continue the rest of the day, and with the aid of a flashlight to illuminate her face, even during her medicated sleep at night.

During that same night, after I had finally finished my work at the hospital and gone home to my apartment in Cambridge, I walked into the bathroom and before I realized what I was doing, had spent a long time just staring at my own face in the mirror. I looked like me, but somehow this was more equivocal, and more comforting, than it had been before.

More than twenty years of practicing psychology have passed since the extremely young intern that I used to be confirmed her own identity in a bathroom mirror. In those years, mostly through much-repeated experience, I have learned to maintain at least the appearance of equanimity when a person, awake and conversational in a room with me, seems to turn into someone else before my very eyes. Certainly, I now know the right things to say and do, and I feel competent, as an experienced therapist, to say and do them. But occasionally, even after all this time, I will still find myself inwardly advising, "Keep breathing, Martha. Remember to breathe . . ." I can now fully appreciate that the potential changeability of our fellow human beings is one of the most daunting aspects of human nature that any of us will ever confront, in a therapy session or anywhere else. And I believe that this is why conspicuous dissociative reactions have been so fascinating to us, and also so repugnant, through the centuries and even to the present day.

More recently than Crystal, one person who has daunted me, and even frightened me once or twice—and also heartened and amazed me more times than I can count—is Garrett. Unlike "Kate" or "Amelia," or Kenneth's anonymous protective shadow, Garrett's dissociated ego states did go around talking to other people, and he was quite clear on this point the very first day he walked into my office.

"Before I say anything else, you need to know that I have MPD," he announced, with the air of someone who knows he may have to leave early should his train be departing.

MPD is the acronym for *multiple personality disorder*, a diagnosis that, in 1994, was renamed *dissociative identity disorder* (DID), in the American Psychiatric Association's *Diagnostic and Statistical Manual of Mental Disorders IV.* The change in terminology reflected a large accumulation of research on trauma and dissociative disorders. For, just as the archaic (and breathtakingly sexist) label of "hysteria" (or "wandering uterus") eventually gave way to a more neutral, objective, and useful list of "anxiety disorders," psychiatric taxonomy may evolve, in the best instances, away from names (like "multiple personality disorder") that reflect dramatic and superstitious cultural notions, toward less provocative, more accurately descriptive diagnoses obtained from research. Such has been the case for dissociative identity disorder.

"You have multiple personality disorder?" I echoed.

"Yes."

"How do you know?"

"Well, I've had five other therapists, and the last three all said I had MPD."

"Oh," I said, as neutrally as I could.

"Do you believe in MPD?" he asked.

"To tell you the truth, I don't think it's really a matter of belief. Dissociative identities just *are*, whether we believe in them or not. Have you ever heard the term 'dissociative identity'?"

"Does the pope live in the woods? I've had five other shrinks, remember?"

"Of course. And the last three 'believed in' dissociative identity disorder?"

"Right."

Though I had hedged a little, Garrett had asked me a legitimate question. Accounts of "multiple personality" have been recorded for more than three hundred years. (In 1646, the Renaissance physician Paracelsus described a woman who was amnesic for an alter ego who stole money from her.) But for various powerful psychological, philosophical, and legalistic reasons, the phenomenon is frightening and downright objectionable to many people. Dissociative identity disorder is the subject of heated disputes in the nonmedical press, which is why Garrett had asked me whether or not I "believed in" it. These controversies presuppose that dissociative identities, like elves or unicorns, are a matter of belief; and based on not much more than strong personal or ideological objections, people often contemptuously disavow DID as fake, doctor-induced (iatrogenic), or the side effect of some tenacious, undiagnosed psychosis. Of particular concern are the questions of personal and legal accountability that the existence of DID is purported to raise.

In addition to being poorly understood, dissociative identity disorder bears the curse of making first-rate American media material. Want a tantalizing segment for your talk show? Try multiple personality disorder. Need a plot twist for your legal thriller? Write in a homicidal multiple. And this entertainment potential has inextricably affected the real people who confront daily nonfictional struggles with their dissociative behavior.

Media attention has influenced the mental health professions as well. DID is not just a diagnosis; it is a badge of honor, a kind of professional plum case. And consequently, some patients will try to fake dissociative identity disorder (to be more interesting to therapists), especially in hospitals and clinics, where diagnoses and the relative amounts of attention they garner are observable by all; sometimes DID is doctor-induced; and probably a small number of misdiagnosed patients are tragically wrestling with psychosis, rather than DID. More commonly, actual dissociative identities revealed by a patient take over the therapy, eclipsing concern for other important aspects of that person's psychological makeup. The revealed ego states are scrutinized, encouraged, elaborated upon by the therapist, instead of being dealt with as what they are—disruptive, often painful products of chronic childhood trauma, that can and should be treated in proportion to their significance.

Emotional embroilments notwithstanding, dissociative identity disorder that has received clinical attention can be systematically investigated using standardized assessment measures. Cross-cultural studies using these instruments, most notably in the United States, the Netherlands, and at the University of Istanbul, demonstrate that patients diagnosed with DID have a stable set of core symptoms throughout North America as well as in Europe and Turkey.

A report from the National Institute of Mental Health states that the "repeated replication of a core clinical phenomenology demonstrates construct validity equal to or superior to that demonstrated for most [psychiatric] disorders." The same report points out, also, that dissociative identity disorder "manifests an historical validity absent in most modern era diagnoses." The existence of DID as a clinical entity constitutes the consensus of medical opinion, and at present, the disorder is studied in major medical centers and traumatic stress research institutes all over the globe, from Belmont, Massachusetts, to Melbourne, Australia.

Yes, I believed in DID.

"I'm definitely the genuine item," Garrett said. "I've got all the credentials. Therapist number five wanted me to write out a list of all my alters. She said she was doing research."

"And did you?"

"No, I didn't. What good would that have done? We didn't get along too well after that, so I left. And that's why I'm here. I mean, I can't just give up. I want to have a *me*."

"What do you mean by 'having a me'?"

"Oh, you know—like the computer people who keep on trying to make a machine with a sense of *I*."

"You don't have a sense of *I*?"

"No. But I have a real big sense of *we*." He chuckled infectiously at his remark.

Garrett, a forty-one-year-old housepainter, was an extraordinarily tall man, just over six and a half feet. He had a poet's features: dark brown curls framed a delicately handsome face set with shining gray eyes and thin, tremulous lips. But by far the dominant aspect of his appearance was his extreme skinniness. His body was so tall and so fleshless, his presentation so mannequinlike, that when he stood, one had the uneasy impression that he was listing, even though he held himself quite straight. In sessions later on, he would tell me that, entirely apart from traumatization or dissociative episodes, some of the saddest events of his childhood involved being teased by other children on account of his bony, stretched-out frame.

There was a subtle languor in Garrett's speech that reminded me of my childhood in the South, but when I asked him where he was from, he said "eastern Long Island."

"When people think of Long Island, they think it has something to do with New York City. But way out in the eastern part, where I'm from, there wasn't much but potato farms. At least, not at the time."

As therapy sessions with him passed, I learned that Garrett's rural childhood had been impossible to bear. When Garrett was five years old, his father was killed in a single-car accident in which suicide was never completely ruled out. The car was demolished when, at high speed, it was driven head-on into a tree. Within a month, Garrett's uncle, his father's oldest brother, moved into the household, and immediately began to terrorize Garrett's mother. According to Garrett, his mother was "pathologically passive her whole life, a poster girl for helpless creatures." The uncle soon began to share her bed; her consent was probably never given, and was in any case, irrelevant to Uncle Dean.

Uncle Dean became Garrett's tormentor, and tormentor of Garrett's baby brother as well. The brother, whose real name I never learned (Garrett referred to him only as "Lef," an unexplained nickname), was four years younger than Garrett, and when his father died, the five-year-old took his one-year-old brother on, as a charge. His mother fed them both, bathed them, washed their clothes; but it was Garrett who kept Lef company, taught him things, kept him out of trouble. Garrett taught Lef to walk, and then to run, and picked him up when he fell. And Garrett tried, without much success, to protect them both from Uncle Dean.

The uncle's controlling and rageful nature directed him to beat the two young boys, viciously and often, for minor and even imagined offenses. One of Garrett's earliest memories, from age seven, was of being injured, and cowering under some bushes where he had been thrown after a beating. On that occasion, he suffered a broken leg, which was not attended to for half a day. In addition, Uncle Dean sexually abused and humiliated Garrett. During therapy, Garrett reported to me that he had a mental picture of being molested by an entire group of men, composed of Dean and Garrett's three other uncles, Dean's remaining brothers. However, Garrett was never certain whether the mental image reflected a real memory or a horrible fantasy.

The most heinous of Uncle Dean's practices was to accuse little Garrett of some wrongdoing, and then to proclaim that, as Garrett's punishment, younger brother Lef, instead of Garrett, was to be hurt. Garrett was required to watch. During one of these proxy beatings, when Lef was six years old, Uncle Dean kicked Lef to death. The uncle was prosecuted, but never convicted, in part because the only witness had been a tall, extra-skinny ten-year-old boy who, eerily, kept insisting that he himself had killed his brother.

After that, Garrett was placed in a series of foster homes, some of them benign, some of them emotionally and sexually abusive.

I remember that when I had heard Garrett's whole story, I said to him quietly, "You are an impressive human being. I don't know how you survived all that. In all honesty, I don't think I would have."

He looked into my eyes for an instant, almost imploringly. But then he looked away and shrugged.

"Yeah, well, some people have it worse," he said.

Garrett's childhood was too terrifying for any child to survive. And so he did not survive it as only one child; he became several children, and these children divvied up the horror, and made it survivable. The several children all lived inside Garrett's head, his various selves. One dissociated ego state was toddlerlike and innocent. One was tough, angry, and sometimes aggressive. The toddler personality called himself "James." The tough guy was "Gordon." There were a few others as well, somewhat amorphous during childhood and adolescence. One of these insistently believed that Garrett had murdered his brother, and should therefore kill himself as well.

Unlike Julia's ego states, who remained hidden even to Julia, Garrett's ego states occasionally replaced him entirely, thought and acted in his stead. But much of the time, Garrett was still Garrett. His behavior was directed by "James" only when he was completely alone, and could feel safe. "Gordon" handled things only when Garrett needed to be physically protected, which happened less frequently as he achieved his superior height. And this system became Garrett's ongoing conscious experience, which he did not question any more than most of us question our ongoing conscious experience. It just was.

Despite his tragic circumstances, he attended a technical high school, and learned house-painting, a task at which he excelled, both in the painting itself, and in terms of habits that enhanced his popularity as a workman: reliability, honesty, a practiced cheerfulness. And of course, people were intrigued by his appearance; they often joked with him that maybe he did not really need a ladder to paint an upper level. Garrett moved to the Boston area during the region's suburban building boom of the 1970s. He persevered at his occupation, and was as proud of his work as if he had been a well-known artist. House-painting had the further advantage of being a job he could do alone, and almost automatically if necessary, making it a living he could conduct through his frequent depressions, and even his bouts of obsessive suicidality. The external activities of his ego states were still rather circumscribed.

He was an intelligent man, an avid reader, humorous despite it all. He taught himself to read and speak Spanish, hoping someday to use his painting skills to help out with Habitat for Humanity, in this country and in Central America. Central America, and its long-suffering populations, fascinated him.

Garrett reluctantly entered his first therapy only because his personalities eventually became hard to control, difficult to "keep in," even when he was in public. Worst of all, they began to come out during work, identifying themselves by name, and attempting to speak with an employer, Frank, whom he particularly liked.

"It was so *embarrassing*," he said to me, covering his eyes with one long, slender hand. And I, of course, thought of Julia. She had been right-on, again.

"I always knew they were there, but I guess I never thought about them very much. They were more or less a private thing, and really, it was only when they started coming out in front of other people, and I saw how people took it—wow!—I knew it was radical, then. But before then, well, there was Garrett and Gordon and James and the others, and that was how it was, and who cared anyway?

"Yeah, now that I think about it, before they really got out of control, I didn't have any reason to see how people reacted. James was always alone, and Gordon, well, he definitely got big reactions, but you figure, who *doesn't* act kind of surprised when somebody sets in to beating them up? And besides, Gordon doesn't really introduce himself. He just sort of takes care of business.

"In fact, you want to hear something funny? This is what I think: I think if names just weren't involved, if alters came out but didn't use their names, most people would still never know. Best example, Frank, my boss—I think if Willie had just come out and acted like Willie, and talked like Willie, but hadn't actually said to Frank, 'Hi, I'm Willie,' Frank wouldn't have blinked. He would have thought—man, that Garrett is weird—and that's about all. Really, I think that's true."

When employer Frank did react, with revulsion, Garrett sought out a therapist. His earnest goal at the time was to keep his alters "in," at least in public. The first therapist gave him the diagnosis of "major depression, recurrent," in a schizotypal personality. She believed that he was having hallucinations. It was not until therapist number three that Garrett's trauma background was recognized, and he was given the more accurate diagnosis of "dissociative identity disorder."

In the *Diagnostic and Statistical Manual of Mental Disorders IV*, "dissociative identity disorder" (diagnosis number 300.14) is defined as the presence of two or more distinct identities or ego states, "each with its own relatively enduring pattern of perceiving, relating to, and thinking about the environment and self," in an individual for whom at least two of these ego states *recurrently take control of behavior.* In addition, the DSM IV specifies, first, that the condition is marked by an "inability to recall important personal information that is too extreme to be explained by ordinary forgetfulness," and second, that the apparent multiplicity of identity is not due to the direct physiological effects of a substance (such as alcohol) or a medical condition (such as complex seizures).

The DSM IV, along with many other research-based sources, states that individuals with DID often report having experienced severe physical and sexual abuse as young children.

These are the core symptoms and associated features of dissociative identity disorder, across cultures. Other signs and characteristics are often, but not universally, observed. Many people with DID, but not all, have the symptoms of post-traumatic stress disorder (exaggerated startle responses, nightmares, flashbacks). Self-mutilation and suicidal or aggressive behaviors may occur. Within the individual, certain ego states and not others may experience psychophysiological phenomena such as pseudoseizures, or a supernormal ability to control pain. And there are reports of marked variations across ego states (within the same individual) in physiological attributes such as visual acuity, asthma symptoms, sensitivity to allergens, and response of blood glucose to insulin. In other words, one personality may be myopic, and the others not so; a certain personality may be asthmatic, and the others free of asthma; and so forth.

The process by which ego states are created and maintained is unknown. The promise of current research is that in the future, we will learn more from psychological and neurobiological studies of how any of us go about forming, consolidating, and recognizing our own identities—beginning with the primitive and mercurial behavioral states of infancy, through the fantasy play and imaginary friends of childhood, and into the relative (but not absolute) stasis of full-fledged, culture-bound adult personalities. All such research will be sorely challenged by the intricacy and authority of the "ego state," which may, among other multiregion properties, include or govern physiological events as fully involuntary as near-sightedness and hypoglycemia.

Ego states that control an individual's behavior may proclaim themselves with proper names, or they may not introduce them-selves at all. Some people with DID realize that they have disso-ciative personalities; many people with DID who are not in therapy—and quite a few who are—do not understand that they are dissociative in this way. Unlike major depression or schizo-phrenia or the flu, DID can be all but invisible, until or unless someone correctly diagnoses it. This fact is, of course, quite con-trary to the popular image of dissociative identity disorder as the conspicuous trademark of raving lunatics. But out in the real world, any of the disorder's symptoms, even the seemingly more remarkable ones such as variations in physiological functioning, can go unnoticed or be misattributed, particularly if alters emerge without proclaiming names for themselves.

Moreover, when symptoms first manifest themselves, calling dissociative identity disorder a "disorder" at all is an equivocal cus-tom. The condition seems to emerge spontaneously in situations of extreme early trauma, and is a highly effective self-protective strategy that may preserve the individual's very life, by allowing him to continue to think and behave *at all* in circumstances that would otherwise be tetanizing. In situations that are too chroni-cally terrifying for the self to deal with, the self may take advantage of its several ego states, may divide the stress, and cope as a group of specialized but interrelated selves. In this way, we survive. In this way, as in so many others, our resilient brains are much more bril-liant than we know.

And Garrett desperately needed "Gordon" and the others, be-cause without them, little Garrett might easily have ceased to be. Alone in circumstances of unremitting fear or grief, in which absolutely nothing can be done, a creature may eventually simply die. This reality has often been naturalistically observed in humans, and experimentally demonstrated with many different species of nonhuman animals, beginning in 1957, when C. P. Richter discovered that healthy wild rats in which "hopelessness" had been experimentally induced often died of parasympathetic arrest of the heart.

Chronically abused children are, in many cases, at genuine risk of dying from protracted uncontrollable stress. But human animals, unlike nonhuman ones, can sometimes use purely psychological coping mechanisms, in the absence of concrete ones. They can dissociate, take a mental vacation from their external reality, as Julia did during much of her childhood; or in conditions of particularly out-of-control and violent physical and sexual abuse, they can call in a mental cavalry of ego states, as Garrett did, and replace themselves entirely. And when these strategies are used to foster survival itself, they must be viewed as adaptive.

By their nature, traumatic circumstances for a young, helpless human often end when that person ceases to be young and helpless, when he grows to adulthood. However, dissociative identities do not shut down in the adult; in fact, they may become more insistent, and when trauma is no longer ongoing, but dissociative identities are still controlling behavior, only then does calling dissociative identity disorder a "disorder" start to make sense. Also, by adulthood, double-edged behavioral tactics intended to numb the suffering, such as drug or alcohol abuse, may have been superimposed on an already too-complicated picture.

Still, particularly if the various ego states do not claim proper names, DID may remain invisible. If an addiction is present, it may become apparent as a problem long before DID, which may be overlooked or misattributed indefinitely. By his own report, Garrett "never thought about" his condition until, at the age of thirty-two, he thoroughly horrified his boss Frank with the revelation that someone named "Willie" was taking turns painting Frank's house.

During Garrett's therapy, I learned that he had a large number of dissociated ego states, many of whom "came out" at times. He and I never counted exactly how many, because it is unlikely that Garrett himself knew all of his alters. The most prominent ones were still "James," who remained a small child, and the defender, "Gordon," who had grown older along with Garrett. In addition, there was the problematic "Willie," a devout, Bible-thumping alter who often went to church on Sundays, despite the fact that Garrett was a nonbeliever. Among the congregation of this church, only "Willie" was known. No one had ever met Garrett; therefore, no one had the first clue that he was dissociative. Then there was the sinister "Abe," the alter who believed that Garrett had killed his younger brother, Lef. Alarmingly to me, this personality sometimes "came out" to insist that justice would not be served by anything less than Garrett's suicide. "Abe" seemed to be the dissociated ego state charged with bearing the shame and pain of Garrett's having witnessed his brother's murder.

Another alter, calling himself "Big James," seemingly a slightly older version of the original "James," would speak occasionally, in a still childlike voice, to express his fear that "Abe" would persuade Garrett to kill himself. "Big James" understood that, if this happened, he, "Big James," would die, too. And "Big James" did not want to die. The struggle between "Big James" and "Abe" was the most striking example of the observation that, in general, Garrett's alters disagreed with each other, and with Garrett, quite a lot.

When Garrett switched to an alter, he lost his observing ego. For example, "Willie" never thought to himself, "Gee, this is not like me. I need to get a grip on myself." Such internal commentary is a function of the observing ego, and Garrett's was lost to him when a dissociated ego state took over. Though temporarily, "Willie" (or "James" or "Abe" or "Gordon") was completely present, and Garrett was altogether absent.

Because therapy for Garrett often involved his remembering Uncle Dean, and others who had abused him in childhood, the angry "Gordon" was the personality triggered most often in therapy

sessions. I met "Gordon" for the first time on a mid-January afternoon, after I had known Garrett for about six months, during a
session in which Garrett was recalling the broken leg he had suffered when he was seven. He had recounted this event in an earlier
session, and on this winter's day was alluding to it again, rather
matter-of-factly, because that morning, while walking in Boston,
he had happened to see a little boy in a leg brace.

"Actually, I don't think he had a broken leg. I think there was
something wrong with his leg, like from birth or something. His
mom was walking along beside him, being real nice to him. I mean,
I couldn't actually hear what she was saying, but she was patting
him and smiling and everything."

Garrett's liquid gray eyes reflected pleasure as he described the
anonymous boy's mother and her kind demeanor. He lounged in
his leather chair, content, with his legs straight out in front of him
in a tremendous letter V. He was wearing the longest, slimmest
navy blue sweat suit I had ever seen, and I wondered to myself once
again how he ever found clothing in a size to fit his extraordinary
form.

"I bet she's a really good mom," he said. Then he was silent for
a moment or two, pensive, until finally he remarked, in a seeming
non sequitur, "It's really cold out there."

Silence again, lengthy enough this time that finally I said, "It's
really cold out there. Something made you think about the cold?"

Garrett did not answer me, and I never discovered what his
thought had been. He stared straight ahead, toward the big double
doors. I watched his face, and as I watched, Garrett became another person, in the space of about twenty seconds. His lips tight-
ened, his brow furrowed, and his large, smiling gray eyes turned
into angry, dry slits, disturbingly backlit. With a speed I would
have thought physiologically impossible, all of the flesh tone left
his skin, which instantly assumed a bloodless taupe color, not quite
human.

When this swift transformation was complete, he immediately
gripped the arms of his chair and propelled himself into a standing

position, all six and a half feet of him. Where Garrett's posture was straight, this person slouched menacingly. He waved his arms in the air, and began to pace in long steps back and forth across my office, from bookshelf to bookshelf.

The change was utterly convincing, and I realized that I had uncharacteristically folded my arms, as if to warm or perhaps protect myself.

"Son of a bitch! Son of a bitch!" he growled.

"Gordon?" I guessed.

He stopped pacing and stared at me for a long moment, as if trying to recognize someone.

"Yeah. Oh, yeah, it's you." He stared for another moment, and then apparently deciding that I was acceptable, resumed his trips across my office.

"Son of a bitch! I should've killed him myself before he had the *chance* to die. Fucking heart attack! I never got the chance. Did you know that? I never got the chance. I should've held that old man down and ripped off his balls and stuffed them in his fucking mouth! I should've fucking killed him myself! I'm a black belt, you know."

Entirely gone was Garrett's soft, languid speech pattern. While "Gordon's" accent was not faultlessly New York, it was closer to the city than to eastern Long Island. And, to be sure, gone was Garrett's scrupulous avoidance of vulgar language.

"Gordon" continued to pace and rave for a full five minutes. My presence in the room seemed almost immaterial. Finally, I politely asked him to stop, and when to my surprise he did so right away, I inquired whether I might speak with Garrett again. Without comment, "Gordon" returned to his chair, sat down, and in the twinkling of an eye fell, to all appearances, fast asleep.

I was breathless.

I let him sleep for a few minutes, and then I quietly called, "Garrett? Garrett, are you there? You need to wake up, Garrett."

His eyes fluttered, and slowly he became awake. The usual color had returned to his face, which was Garrett's once more.

He looked at me questioningly, and I said, "Welcome back."

"Oh no," he said softly, and covered his face with his hands.

I talked with Garrett, who was mortified to have switched in my presence, about how much he had needed "Gordon" when he was younger, about how "Gordon" had helped to save his life, psychologically, and perhaps literally on some occasions. I suggested that someday "Gordon" could be greatly modified and integrated as a protective part of Garrett's own personality. But on that day, Garrett remained unhappy, and far beyond skeptical.

Later on, as I thought about this session, I reflected upon a detail—that "Gordon" had claimed to be a black belt, presumably in one of the martial arts. I recalled the number of times I had heard the tough-guy ego states of various people speak of being black belts, always using the particular term "black belt," and I visualized battalions of dissociated ego states, male and female, enrolled in martial arts classes across the country, something like "Willie" going to church on Sundays. The notion of a "black belt" as the ultimate in survival-readiness has been instilled in our cultural consciousness to such an extent that any personality developing within our society, dissociated or not, will see it that way. And so, if you are a protector personality, desperately needing to be ready for anything and anyone at all times, you should be a "black belt," without a doubt.

I wondered whether "Gordon" had taken instruction, or was just boasting, but I shall never know. Such an actual question would be too incendiary for the volatile "Gordon." In either case, our cultural fascination with Bruce Lee movies, and breaking bricks with our bare hands, had left its imprint. "Gordon" was clearly a late-century American.

Cultural influences shape dissociative identity disorder all over the planet. For example, in cultures where spirit possession figures large in prevailing belief systems, dissociated ego states may be perceived as spirits entering from the outside, rather than as resident alter egos. That cultural differences affect the perceived locus of an identity disturbance is supported by research in India, South

Asia, and China. "Possession" patients in the Hebei province of China bearing the diagnosis of *yi-ping* (hysteria) manifest symptoms impressively similar to those displayed by DID patients in the American state of Massachusetts. And in this very country, when religious exorcisms are performed upon those believed to have been entered by Satan, these rites almost certainly involve individuals with DID, perhaps primarily so.

Perceptions are strongly influenced by situational as well as cultural factors. When Garrett's antisocial behavior began, I was sitting in a therapy room with him, and therefore I perceived him, and dealt with him, in a particular way. I knew that he had dissociative identity disorder. I knew, because he had told me so, that he had a fierce, angry ego state named "Gordon." And so, when he abruptly became angry and fierce, I surmised that "Gordon" had just taken over his thoughts and actions. But what if, without calling himself by name, "Gordon" were to take over while Garrett was amidst a group of uninitiated strangers, or even acquaintances? How would they know that Garrett was dissociative? The answer is, of course, that they probably would not know. They might be appalled by him, or frightened of him. They might say that he was bizarre. If they had to deal with him on a continuing basis, they would "walk on eggshells" around him, and discuss him behind his back. But, most likely, they would not realize that he had dissociative identity disorder. DID is too exotic. DID is supposed to be the property of mental hospitals, and television.

They might react similarly—huge astonishment, perhaps fear, curiosity, and gossip—should he switch to a whimpering child, or an insistent religious proselytizer, or a withdrawn fanatic brooding upon suicide; but they probably would not say, "Aha! Dissociative identity disorder."

I have seen florid DID be completely unrecognized in a crowd. As an illustration, I recall an unexpected New Year's Day snowstorm in Washington, D.C., which paralyzed that southerly city, so cosmopolitan, and so charmingly unequipped to deal with eight inches of snow. I was at Washington National Airport, trying to get home, along with throngs of other sleepy-eyed people who had finished their New Year's Eve celebrations. My flight was just about to board when Washington National Airport closed down entirely, due to weather conditions. Exasperating, but an act of God. Turning from the gate, trying to formulate a new plan, I slowly became aware of a conversation, gaining in volume, between an airline representative at the desk, and a customer. It went something like this:

"The airport is closed, sir. No one can get in or out, on account of the storm."

"I have to get on that plane. Open the door."

"Sir, the entire airport is closed. All flights are canceled."

"No. I have to get on that plane. Let me pass."

The man was expensively dressed, in a banker's suit, and he would not be dissuaded. He got louder. He got so loud that people began to turn back toward the gate to watch him. A second airline representative joined the situation. The man, who had turned ashen in the face, waved his fists at the two representatives, and shrieked at them to let him get on the plane. By now, the man had the attention of at least a hundred strangers, who had stopped in their tracks to stare at his outrageous behavior. He continued to scream his demand. Security was called. Three uniformed men arrived, took the elegant fellow in tow, and hauled him off, still ranting.

People muttered nervously to one another, and then went on their way. I believe very few of them knew what they had just witnessed. Though they could have described it well, they would not have labeled it accurately. "Control freak," I heard someone in the crowd explain, a conception as familiar in our culture as is spirit possession in provincial China. The man's dramatically symptomatic dissociative identity disorder was unrecognized, a reminder to me that to elevate something to the radically exotic is to make it invisible, even—or maybe especially—when it is in plain sight.

It is important to us that dissociative identity disorder be exotic, airily marginal, perhaps even a myth. DID seems to defy so many of our ideas about ourselves as clearly demarcated, self-directed

units, and raises dangerous questions about free will and accountability. ("Oh no, Your Honor. I didn't rob the liquor store. My evil
twin Fred, *he* robbed the liquor store.") But in the chapters that
follow, we will discover that the incidence of dissociative identity
disorder is much greater than is usually understood. And, just as it
is more than possible to operate in the world with a single, constant identity while evincing no notion of accountability at all, it is
possible also to have a deeply bewildering identity disorder that exists simultaneously with a committed sense of responsibility. We
will find that this sense of personal responsibility may well be the
only answer to the elusive riddles posed by the age-old, survival-
focused mental machinery that resides in us all.

In this regard, some of Garrett's remarks about his own identity
disturbance are intriguing. From time to time, I would question
Garrett about the activities and interrelations of his dissociated
ego states. I did not spend excessive amounts of time doing so, because being dissociative was only a part of who Garrett was; Garrett was a complex person, like any other, and deserved to be
treated as such, particularly in his therapy. He had other problems.
His trauma history was unfathomable. He drank straight vodka out
of brimming iced tea glasses, daily. Too often, he avoided social
contact because he was miserably self-conscious about his unusual
physique. And Garrett had impressive strengths, too. He had
steady work that he liked. He was intelligent, engaging, and remarkably humorous. And, like anyone else, he had dreams. He
imagined traveling to Central America, using his skills to help
long-oppressed people build houses for their families.

Recall his entire humanness as you consider the strange-sounding
answers to these specific questions about his dissociative dilemma.
Bear in mind, also, that—for anyone—perhaps nothing defines
unified personhood so solidly as the courage of strong commitment to personal responsibility. Garrett could so easily have
claimed to be *non compos mentis,* with gigantic believability and
reams of medical records to back him up. But he never made that
claim. Instead, as you will see here, he was dedicated to the defin-

ing feature of responsibility for his actions, regardless of which ego state had performed them. And for that reason, I had already begun to think of him as someone who might, quite possibly, recover:

QUESTION: "When did you first realize that you had dissociative personalities?"

ANSWER: "When my third therapist told me so. No, no, that's not fair. I got the label from her, but I already knew the others were in there, even though I didn't think about the whole thing very much. I remember one time when I was about twelve or thirteen—maybe this was the first time, I don't know—I was sitting on my bed, all curled up, sucking my thumb, because James had just left, and when I came back, I took a look around, and I thought, 'Oh boy, this is really strange.' But I didn't have a name for it or anything, not until much later. And besides, I didn't know anything about other people then. For all I knew, other people switched around just like me."

QUESTION: "Is there one personality that's the 'real' you?"

ANSWER: "I don't know."

QUESTION: "Do all of your personalities remember the same life, have the same memories?"

ANSWER: "No, not even close. I don't think James remembers much of anything. He'll always be a child. Gordon remembers the fights, and the really bad times. Willie remembers Sundays, mostly, and a few other times. And me, well, I'm not really sure what I remember."

QUESTION: "Do your personalities know one another?"

ANSWER: "Some of them do. James and Big James know each other, and they know Gordon, because he watches out for them. But Willie doesn't know anyone, except me, of course. And Abe is really a lone wolf. Big James knows him, but Little James doesn't. And I think there may be more of them, ones that even I don't know."

QUESTION: "Do they have conversations with each other in your head?"

ANSWER: "Constantly, constantly, constantly. Sometimes I'd do almost anything to drown them out. Sometimes the vodka helps. What they argue about mainly is that they all want to come out all the time. Like here, with you, right this very second, James is whining and whining and begging to come out. He thinks you're nice, motherly or something. He wants to come out just about every time we're here. And Gordon. Gordon wants to be out because he thinks he's the only one who knows how to deal. He thinks the rest of us can't take care of things. Willie wants to convert me, and everyone in the world, for that matter. He's an unbelievable pain. And Abe. You know about Abe. He wants to die. He talks to me a lot. It's really hard to keep him in. Sometimes I think I can't do it. He wants me to stop coming here, you know."

QUESTION: "Could one of your personalities simply take over all the others at some point?"

ANSWER: "I don't think so. No, I don't think so, not for longer than a few days, anyway. I mean, even Garrett can't do that, right?"

QUESTION: "Could one of them, say, buy a car, or have a friend or a lover the others disliked?"

ANSWER: "Sure. Sometimes I get strange messages on my answering machine from people I don't know. I have CDs that I hate. I have no idea how I got them. Sure."

QUESTION: "What if one of your personalities did something really bad—committed a crime, perhaps—who is responsible in that case?"

ANSWER: "I am."

QUESTION: "Wait a minute. I thought you didn't have a sense of *I*."

ANSWER: "Doesn't matter. I am."

CHAPTER SEVEN

Switchers

The very greatest mystery is in unsheathed reality itself.
—Eudora Welty

Grandma Cleopatra, once a motherless "wee trouper," and now a sixty-six-year-old woman—is she a frightening person? If we had been standing in the room with her when she first picked up her grandson, and if we could have read her mind to know that, at such an emotional moment, she felt absolutely nothing—that in fact she was dissociated from a part of her own self—would we have been scared of her? Would our pupils have dilated in alarmed fascination with this silver-haired lady and her behavior?

Probably not.

Triggered by current anxieties that called up decades-old childhood calamities and impossible struggles with her grade-school brothers, she was detached from a portion of her reality when she met her first grandchild, and being detached from reality is a functional definition of insanity. Standing in that room, would we have viewed her as temporarily insane, and perhaps snatched the baby from her?

Not likely.

We would not see Cleo as insane, even temporarily—or Kenneth, or Laura, or Matthew, or ourselves—and we would not be even remotely frightened or fascinated, because although we formally define sanity as the state of being in touch with reality, our actual images of sanity have little to do with mental and behavioral groundedness. Rather, our images of sanity are constructed almost exclusively from our ongoing judgments of *behavioral acceptability and consistency*. Cleo may be as detached from her own emotions as Jupiter is from Earth, but as long as she continues to behave acceptably and consistently, like a grandmother, the issue of her sanity will never be even a blip in anyone else's thoughts.

Kenneth, the father who is afraid of heights, may struggle with darkly paranoid thoughts, reaching the magnitude of clinical significance, sparked by his tormented (and dissociated) childhood in a bigoted neighborhood; but as long as he retains his observing ego and continues to direct his behavior, at least in the major ways, like Kenneth always has, no one will express even the tiniest interest in the integrity of his mental status.

The demifugue state of Laura, the college student with the alcoholic family, feels and looks like sleepiness. And though the occurrence of four days of sudden, impenetrable fatigue in a rested nineteen-year-old is improbable in the extreme—unless it be a bright red flag for some medical problem—every person around Laura during a crowded Thanksgiving holiday will readily accept sleepiness as an adequate explanation for her behavior.

And Matthew the space cadet—well, Matthew is a little more problematic, because he sometimes causes trouble for others, and worse, his behavior is inconsistent. Most of the time, he is an attentive, articulate professional type; every now and then, he is seemingly the opposite, spaced-out, unresponsive. But the uncomfortable question of Matthew's groundedness in reality is neatly circumvented by his friends, and by his wife, who provide him with identities that are stock and portable, even if not entirely flattering: "absentminded professor," "coward."

All of us work extremely hard to see consistency in other people, and in ourselves as well. Because we are so inextricably dependent upon one another, especially upon our mates, our parents, and our friends—and because everyone knows that human beings are, with no close second, the most dangerous species on the planet—we desperately wish to believe that people are calculable quantities, consistent and therefore predictable. We want to know what to expect from them, and we want to know it every time. Some even hold fast to a belief, despite overwhelming evidence to the contrary, that beyond merely predicting their fellows, they can control them, as well.

Because the general predictability of those near to us is of such excruciating importance to a sense of safety in our lives, we eagerly provide, or agree with, explanatory labels, complicated rationalizations, outrageous excuses, and mind-bending psychological hypotheses, when confronted by apparent inconsistencies. We are impressively creative, and sometimes ridiculous, in these endeavors, which are intended to wrap up otherwise baffling arrays of dissimilar behaviors into packages that we can put knowable handles on, with philosophical tape and bobby pins if we have to.

For Matthew's friends, the tacit, unspoken process went something like this: We, his friends, see that sometimes Matthew is smart and sociable; sometimes he is spacey and mute. He is inconsistent and therefore unpredictable, and this state of affairs is unacceptable. But wait. What kind of a person goes back and forth between intelligence and stupor? Why, an absentminded professor, of course. There! Problem solved.

Psychology itself, sometimes defined as "the science of prediction and control," has historically been blindsided by this phenomenon among its human subjects. Most frustrated has been the subspecialty of *personality assessment*, which is the branch of psychology that attempts to study personality traits—such as absentmindedness—and also introversion, extraversion, passivity, aggressivity, generosity, greed, competitiveness, empathy, and so forth, into quite a long list.

In traditional personality studies, raters try to infer how much of a given trait a person "has" by observing that person in a laboratory. But in a classic text called *Personality and Assessment*, originally published in 1968, researcher and theorist Walter Mischel showed us that personality traits are mostly suppositions on the part of the laboratory observer, rather than real attributes of the person who is observed. And since 1968, psychologists have discovered that people will, quite involuntarily, misperceive or grossly distort facts in order to achieve a view of others and of themselves that is *consistent*. A number of cognitive and perceptual processes collude in our brains to assist us in doing so.

This does not necessarily mean that personality traits do not exist. But it does mean that we often imagine them when they are not there.

As an illustration of how consistency can be attributed rather than real—and of how crucial consistency is to us—let us refer back to Kenneth. Kenneth is usually a good-humored individual, but his fearful visit to the World Trade Center enlivened an angry dissociated ego state that intruded but did not take over. On the evening after the father-and-son outing, should Kenneth's wife notice the changes in his behavior (her normally warm and approachable husband is now dour and avoidant), she will likely explain these to herself by thinking they are the predictable reactions to something objectionable she has done. She will be more than willing to implicate herself, rather than see her own husband as unpredictable. Or, since she has known for a long time about his "secret" fear of heights, perhaps she will get marginally closer to the truth, and think that he has wound up in a temporary "bad mood" on account of his recent adventure.

If Kenneth's protective ego state begins to erupt much more often, his wife may eventually change her mind about her once even-tempered spouse, and start to think of him as a generally "moody" person. Her official view of Kenneth will then be that he is predictably "moody," rather than predictably even-tempered. But still, he is consistent, if only consistently moody. He is her husband Kenny. Never will she see him as fragmented within himself, and therefore fundamentally inconsistent.

Now imagine that Kenneth is a more profoundly traumatized person than anyone realized, least of all Kenneth himself. Let us grimace and say that, in addition to being hounded as the "Russian kid" in his community, he was also the victim of chronic sexual abuse in his own home. In this even sadder account, Kenneth loses the strong *observing ego* he retained in the original story, such that he does not, or cannot, even try to conduct himself like Kenneth when a dissociated ego state intrudes. His wife, in this version, will be thrown into an almost unbearable turmoil. The anxiety level of her entire life will increase, for she will discover over time that her own husband is inconsistent beyond her ability to discount. Sometimes he is warm, wonderful, and optimistic, and sometimes he is suspicious and rageful. He is much more than "moody"; this man seems like two different people altogether.

Nervously, and often angrily, she will do and say everything she can think of to turn him into the person she imagines to be Kenneth. She will be certain that there is something about this situation she simply has not figured out yet, and that if she can just determine what it is, everything will make sense. She may even joke uneasily with others about her husband's "multiple personalities," never understanding that this is not a joke. Without his observing ego, Kenneth could be diagnosed with a full-blown dissociative identity disorder (DID).

For a long while, years perhaps, Kenneth's wife will try to make him behave consistently like Kenneth; she will try to find the explanation, labor to dredge up some answer. Her endeavors will be cruelly encouraged by the fact that sometimes Kenneth will go for weeks or even months without switching. When she finally does abandon her search, she may divorce him. Or, just as likely, she may remain unhappily married to him, because hope springs eternal in on-again, off-again situations. (Maybe the Kenneth she loves will come back to stay!) She herself may become chronically anxious, or depressed. But she will never seriously consider that her husband (or her ex-husband) has the scary and "rare disease" of dissociative identity disorder. Such a complete realization would give the defining shove to her already precarious understanding of the world and its limits.

The only event that might transform her into an accurate diagnostician would be that in which one of Kenneth's dissociated ego states overtly introduced itself to her, using a proper name (e.g., an ego state were to pipe up and say to her, "Hello. I'm Ivan."). If this happened, she might very well have a sudden, horrified insight, and begin to make a lot of frantic phone calls to professionals. But this clarifying event will probably never occur. Kenneth's ego states may not consciously have proper names, and they may not be sufficiently aware of themselves as multiple entities ever to go about introducing themselves so directly.

Trying to deal with this kind of Kenneth, his spouse is trapped in a destructive psychological riddle from which there is no means of escape, apart from the plain, but life-altering truth. And it is unlikely that she will ever choose such a dark and spooky door, regardless of how anxious or depressed she may become. We do not like explanations that tilt the universe, even when they are answers that might save our lives.

Just like Kenneth's wife, we all have a compelling need to believe that people are unitary and consistent—a need that, if necessary, we will defend by subverting our own most accurate perceptions. And this need is exactly why someone like my patient Garrett—unlike Kenneth or Grandma Cleo—is decidedly alarming and fascinating to most of us, including those of us who are psychotherapists. Someone like Garrett absolutely prevents us from using our imaginative abstractions to explain, and thereby feel safe with, his utterly inconsistent behavior. He does announce, without qualification, that he has several different personalities, and that each of these personalities has a proper name. They will not be lumped together in some clumsy conceptual package to which we can affix a calming, unifying label. They are several, and they will think and behave severally. Such an explicit announcement, coming as it does from a single biological entity with but one face, head, and body, sends us all reeling from a sense of radical other-worldliness.

But we are spellbound precisely because we dimly sense that, in truth, this may be the world where we have been living all along.

In our world, our usual, everyday world, a significant portion of the general population is composed of switchers, people whose personal histories include severe trauma, underestimated abuse or some other grim situation, that has taken them beyond simple dissociative absences, into the realm of dissociative identity disorder. That we do not commonly understand this fact is due mostly to a natural, safety-seeking wish not to see, along with a mistaken cultural belief that all people with dissociative identity disorder openly call themselves by dozens of different names, and tend to be housed in locked wards.

Since about forty-seven out of every one thousand American children are reported as victims of child abuse, using only child abuse as our basis—and no more than those cases of abuse that are actually reported to agencies—we can estimate that nearly five percent of Americans, almost one in twenty people, have histories that could readily generate dissociated ego states, many of these states powerful enough to overwhelm the stabilizing function of the observing ego. The form of dissociative identity disorder in which the "alters" overtly call themselves by different names has been shown to be uncommon; most studies point to less than one percent of the population for this dramatic form of the disorder. But dissociative identity disorder in which the various ego states do not identify themselves is relatively ordinary. Just like the rest of us, most people with DID call themselves by only one name. And, by far, most people with DID will never be therapy patients, let alone inmates on mental wards.

In fact, Nathan was a psychiatrist himself. When I first met him as a colleague, he was approaching forty, and his career was blossoming. He was handsome, financially enviable, and had scores of "friends," people who would smile and say "great guy" when his name was mentioned, but who never seemed to know very much about him, really, apart from the conspicuous trappings of his growing success, and the consensus that he was "entertaining to be around."

This aura of mystery was not a product of Nathan's keeping to himself. Quite the contrary, he was an extraordinarily sociable person. He reveled in parties, attended as many professional conferences as he could, remembered everyone's birthday, and was always the first to suggest get-togethers after work. He excelled at social athletics; in a certain "mood," he was, by unanimous acclaim, almost supernaturally unbeatable at handball.

Nor did he reside by himself. Nathan lived with his wife of fifteen years, and their two children.

And the mysteriousness did not come from his being obviously private, either; rather, he seemed more than willing to share facts about his past, often including facts that were intimate and startling. These self-disclosures from him were presented always as if they were macabre entertainments for the listener, and Nathan himself would laugh heartily at them, closing his stories with commentary such as "Isn't that the weirdest thing you've ever heard?" Surprisingly, the stories often did entertain people—Nathan was a good storyteller—though listening to him was sometimes vaguely eerie.

For example, the very week we were introduced, Nathan told me of an incident from his childhood that was intensely personal and sad, and he related this story in an amused and entirely casual fashion. It seems that when he was about five years old, Nathan's mother ("my crazy mother") discovered him innocently inspecting his own erect penis, whereupon she flew into an all-consuming rage. Screaming at him that he was dirty and evil, she whirled around his bedroom and grabbed up some pairs of his small dungarees that were folded on a chair. With the pants in one hand and Nathan's wrist clamped in the other, she marched with him outside to the backyard barbecue, threw the clothing onto the grill, doused the cloth with lighter fluid, and set it ablaze. When his pants were ashes, and when she had done bawling about the wicked little boy, for all the neighbors to hear, she sent him back to his room until the next morning.

Shaking his head and smiling, and in a hail-fellow-well-met sort of way, Nathan asked me, "Isn't that the weirdest thing you've ever heard?"

To be honest, especially given the nature of my profession, this was not the weirdest thing I had ever heard. However, the story was exceptionally sad, and I understood that, awful as it was, it probably represented only the conscious tip of an unfathomed iceberg, where terrors in this man's childhood had been concerned.

No, the sense of mystery around Nathan did not derive from his being discreet about his history. The pervasive impression that no one really knew anything about him came instead from his unwavering emotional detachment, seemingly from everything, including most particularly his own past. He never revealed his heart, and one could have known his complete autobiography, in great detail, and still Nathan the human being would have been unknown. The man, with all his stories, was an attractive enigma, an emotional blank screen.

In this regard, he could be said to have chosen his profession well, one in which the practitioner is often required to leave his own emotions at the door, so to speak, and immerse himself for an hour in the emotional conundrums of another. Still, Nathan was different. At the end of the working hour, there were no personal feelings waiting by the door for this therapist. He never reassumed his own defining internal life, but rather seemed to have divested his feelings in some much more permanent fashion. I believe that some colleagues and friends may have mistaken this for strength, may even have envied it, as perfect self-containment or invulnerability on Nathan's part, rather than recognizing this characteristic as a lifelong emotional compartmentalization that dangerously exceeded his ability to direct it.

Adding to his aura of elusiveness was Nathan's tendency to be a no-show at events, sometimes events that he himself had organized, and sometimes even long-standing patient appointments. His patients adored him, and so they accepted his unreliability. His secretary often remarked that he was a great guy, but someday he would drive her to leap out a window.

A formal party given by Nathan, and held at his offices, was legendary for his having not attended it at all, nor could he be located by his secretary for the entire weekend that followed the gala. This occurrence was referred to as "outrageous," and "just like him." A few people were angry; most were amused and intrigued. But when he came back to work on Monday, Nathan would not say where he had been. In fact, inquiries put to Nathan about his no-shows most often got a blank expression, almost as if he could not understand why people were questioning him. Or sometimes he would look bemused, make a brief, transparent excuse, and then go on as if nothing had happened. And again, people seemed a little envious of this man, who seemingly was not always bound by social conventions, and who, by their interpretation, was so "independent" that he would not supply explanations for his behavior.

On a number of occasions, Nathan and his wife, Melissa, invited me to dinner at their home, which was large and stylish, and set up for frequent entertaining. During after-dinner coffee, out of the same curiosity felt by nearly everyone who knew him, I would often steer the conversation to the subject of Nathan himself. On one evening in particular, his wife was quite forthcoming, almost as if she had long wished for the opportunity to speak openly with someone on the topic. I had asked her about her husband's no-shows and absences. Did Nathan behave the same way toward his own family? And did this behavior not give her ulcers?

"Ulcers?" Melissa answered. "Let me tell you that I single-handedly finance the production of Tagamet. Sometimes he'll disappear for a whole day and night, or even longer. When I see him again, he acts as if nothing has happened. If I ask him any questions about it, he just looks surprised, actually *surprised*, and then if I really push him to explain, he'll say he was away at some conference or something, out of town. 'I thought I told you about that,' he'll say. Or sometimes he'll say that he went down to the vacation house, to take a 'breather' for a while. And these 'breathers' are sacred. If I complain about them, or ask about them at all, he gets really angry, I mean nuclear-blast angry. He does everything for everybody all the time, he says, and sometimes he just needs to go off by himself. Because he takes care of so many people, he deserves to go off by himself whenever he feels like it, according to him.

"I'd think he was having affairs, except he just doesn't act like I imagine a womanizer does. He's really loving with me. He never has slick excuses all lined up, in fact completely the opposite. I've never gotten suspicious phone calls, or any signs of other women. No, I think he's completely faithful. He just . . . he just disappears sometimes."

I was seated in an overstuffed armchair in the couple's plush living room, and Melissa and Nathan had taken comfortable spots at opposite ends of a huge sectional sofa. When Melissa expressed her belief in his fidelity, Nathan stood and relocated himself next to his pretty wife. Looking extremely happy, he gave her a big hug, and a kiss on the ear.

"You know me so well," he said. And then pointing at Melissa's delicate chin, he said to me earnestly, "This is the only lady for me. She knows my heart and soul."

He waited for Melissa to smile at his statement, and then he stood again and headed for the kitchen. He seemed not in the least disturbed or embarrassed by her account of his disappearances, nor by the fact that she was relating this rather personal information to me. If anything, like a little boy, he looked pleased that the two of us were spending so much time talking about him.

By the time he returned, carrying a tray with fresh coffee and an assortment of Italian chocolates, Melissa and I were involved in our conversation again. I was asking about her two children, ten and eight years old. Did they notice their father's behavior?

"The kids accept whatever their father does," Melissa explained. "They adore him—he's really a great dad, very involved—and I try to act calm around them when I don't know where Nathan is. Of course, sometimes they get disappointed, if we've planned something special for them, and he doesn't show up. But for the most part, they just accept whatever happens. Of course, they're still young, and I worry about when they get older—about whether or not they'll feel demeaned or something when he stands them up. I mean, well, it feels demeaning to *me*, to tell you the truth."

There was a conspicuous pause while she studied Nathan's face, as if trying to gauge the extent of his tolerance. She seemed to want to say more. Nathan was pouring coffee, and still appeared relaxed and cheerful, the good host. Melissa's feet had been tucked under her as she sat on the sofa, and now she shifted her position, planting her feet on the floor.

Returning her gaze to me, she said, "But the things I really worry about are the jealous rages."

"Jealous rages? *Moi?*" interjected Nathan in mock surprise.

Melissa gave a small, nervous laugh.

"Jealous rages?" I asked.

"It's unbelievable sometimes," she continued. Nathan was still jovial, and she evidently felt emboldened to tell me more. "It could be something from a long time before we were married, something from when I was a kid. Let me think of an example . . . Yes, well, the most recent time was when we were up in Montreal for the weekend, just the two of us, about a month ago, wasn't it?"

She glanced at Nathan, who smiled at her and nodded, and then she went on, "Yes, about a month ago. We were having a really good time. We had dinner at Les Halles—I remember we were sharing a *Paris-Brest* for dessert, this beautiful puff pastry with praline creme inside—have you ever had one?—and I don't even remember what we were talking about, but all of a sudden, out of the clear blue sky, he said to me, 'Did you ever eat here with Brian?' Now, Brian was a kid I went out with when I was in college. I spent a summer in Montreal, after my freshman year, and I met a kid named Brian there, and we palled around for a while, until we both had to go back to school. A long, long time ago, before I knew about the jealousy thing of course, I made the big mistake of telling Nathan about that summer, and other stuff about the past, and wow do I regret that. What horror scenes he throws!"

"Horror scenes?" I asked, looking at Nathan. He shrugged.

Melissa answered, "Yes, truly. I say, 'Nathan, don't start.' But by the time I can get that much out, he's already gone. And there's no getting him back. It sort of has a life of its own. His whole face changes—you'd hardly recognize him—and just like that, bang, he's living, breathing rage. I've tried reasoning, pleading, crying. *Nothing* works. I might as well be talking to a wall. That night in Montreal, he went on and on, asking me all kinds of just nonsense questions about some girlhood boyfriend I don't even think about anymore, except when Nathan brings him up. 'Have you talked to Brian recently? Is Brian as smart as me?' On and on, in this awful, hateful voice, not even Nathan anymore. I tell you, it's spooky. That night, I started to cry, right there in the restaurant. He didn't even notice. You can't imagine how embarrassed I was."

She paused and took a breath. Nathan, who had begun to look at her with concerned tenderness in his face, moved next to her again and stroked her hair.

"You're my angel, Melissa," he said gently. And then suddenly grinning, he added, "And besides, I'll bet old Brian couldn't afford *Les Halles*. Am I right?"

She met his eyes briefly. "Lunatic," she scoffed, half playful, half sincere.

Then to me she said, "Do you see that? Sometimes he's perfectly okay with the very same thing that sets him off other times.

Now you're going to think I'm the crazy one. But I tell you, Martha, sometimes he turns into someone I'll bet you wouldn't know if you met him on the street."

"These jealous rages, to use your expression, how do they end?" I asked.

"I'd say they just end by themselves. That's why I said they have lives of their own. Or at least, I've never found anything that I can say or do to get him back when he's in one. He rages like that for a while, and then he usually gets into a thing where he won't speak at all. Icy-cold shoulder—I might as well be furniture. That night in Montreal, later, basically I was trapped in a hotel room with someone I didn't even know, and who acted as if I weren't there. I remember that he lay down on the bed with all his clothes on, finally, and just went to sleep. Slept like a baby all night, peaceful as you please. Of course, I couldn't sleep a wink. I couldn't even close my eyes. And then in the morning, when he woke up, he was fine. He was Nathan again. And he acted as if nothing had happened, I swear, as if nothing had happened. I was too scared to say anything about it, because I couldn't handle any more, and he just started his day, just exactly as if *nothing* had happened. I remember we got ready and went down to Sunday brunch at the hotel, like Dr. and Mrs. Perfectly Fine."

Observing Nathan, I saw that he was listening in more or less the same attitude as myself, as someone who was hearing about something for the first time. And amazingly, to all outward appearances, he was still entirely unoffended by the conversation.

"And that's another thing," Melissa continued. "He has the world's most convenient memory. In fact, maybe this is the most unbearable thing of all. Sometimes when I ask him to discuss all this with me, the things I've been telling you, he'll say he doesn't know what I'm talking about, and then he'll ask me for an example, and when I give him one, he'll just say it never happened. I'll give him a specific incident, exactly when it happened, exactly where we were, what I said, what he said—and then he'll tell me that it never happened, and he doesn't know what I'm talking about. He says it with such *conviction*. Makes me feel like I'm losing my mind, or somebody's doing some kind of sadistic experiment on me, or something. It would be as if, maybe, you called me tomorrow and thanked me for dinner, and I said, 'What dinner?' and then I told you that you hadn't been here, and I didn't have the slightest idea what you were talking about. It would make you nuts, right?"

"Right," I responded.

"I wish you wouldn't do that, Nathan. If you don't want to discuss something with me, just tell me that. Don't say it didn't happen. That makes me nuts. It's a whole lot worse than just refusing to talk."

"I'm sorry, angel," he replied in agreement. "I won't do it again."

There was a silence, during which I decided to try putting on my clinician's hat:

"Nathan, doesn't it bother you that you lose time?"

Dismissively waving both hands at me, he quipped, "Hey! No shop talk here."

Seeing this reaction, Melissa changed her tone. "Oh dear. I think I must be making my own husband sound like a beast. He's not, you know. He's actually wonderful. He's brilliant, he's funny, he's generous, he's a great dad—he's everything anyone could want. It's just that . . . well, I guess even the best of us have our moments."

And after that, the subject soon changed to the far less threatening topic of how much we all liked to visit Montreal.

As a result of these social evenings at Melissa and Nathan's house, I began to think of Nathan as a particularly striking unacknowledged case of dissociative identity disorder. His case seems special if only because he was an unrecovered trauma survivor who presumably treated other unrecovered trauma survivors, with what degree of success I really am not sure. I do know that his patients loved him, and appeared to forgive him his unprofessional lapses.

Of course, there remains the question of why Melissa forgave him. Why does anyone continue in an intimate relationship with someone who is many? At one point in another conversation, and in Nathan's absence, I had the opportunity to approach this question, though I did so rather obliquely.

"With all this unpredictability, don't you get pretty tired?"

Melissa, in reply, was a good deal more direct. "You mean why do I stay?"

"Well yes. I guess I do mean that."

She laughed, and then she said, "My husband is the most complicated person I've ever known. He's also the most energetic, the most intense, and the most fascinating. By a landslide. He does wonderful things, wonderful, adventurous things that no one else does, at least not in real life. It's sort of hard to explain."

"So give me an example. Sounds wonderful."

"It is wonderful. I mean, some of the time it's wonderful. And some of the time it's unbearable."

She looked bemused.

"Okay," she continued, brightening. "An example. We go night-skiing. I don't mean at one of those downhill night-skiing places, with the floodlights. I mean that when the moon is full, sometimes Nathan and I go out with the cross-country skis, and we find a beautiful place, and we ski. Oh, and then there was that time when I happened to mention, just in passing, that I'd love to see Carnival in Trinidad someday. It was the next week. The *next week*, mind you. Before I knew what was happening, there were four plane tickets to Trinidad—I remember it was the week of the March school break—I don't know what kind of magic he used—and when we got there, he had costumes for us, even Benjamin, who was I think five at the time."

She shook her head and laughed again. "I just remembered—he had a little Toulouse-Lautrec costume for Ben—it was hysterical! And so we didn't just see Carnival in Trinidad, we were in it, all of us. It was amazing! And the kids will never, never forget it, of course."

She was silent then. She looked down, and her smiling face slowly turned sad.

After a moment, she said, "But then there are the nightmares, I mean the waking nightmares. All of a sudden, he'll just turn into someone I don't recognize at all. Or he'll disappear, and I never really know how long it's going to be, and . . . and you know, you can really believe me—there is nothing on the face of this earth that a person can do to make you feel more insignificant, less . . . loved—more like you're really less than nothing to him, *less than nothing*—than disappearing on you, just going away. No matter what your plans were, or your children's. No matter how much you needed him. It just doesn't matter. . . .

"I get frightened. It's hard to explain. Not the usual kind of frightened—it's existential fright, or some such thing. He's gone, and I try to picture him in my mind's eye, and the face I see scares me. And then I feel like maybe I don't have the first idea who this man really is. I've been married to him for nearly sixteen years, I sleep with him every night . . . well, nearly every night . . . and he could be anyone in the world. He could just be anyone, and I really wouldn't know."

Another pause, and then, almost to herself, "I don't know anyone else like Nathan. I'm sure I never will. He's wonderful, you know."

Melissa seemed aggrieved as she made this claim, and I felt great sympathy for her. And I could see she was not going to leave Nathan, would probably never leave him, because the brilliance of the man, his uncanny ingenuity at living, mesmerized her. Her life with Nathan, the on-again, off-again of it, the edgy excitement of it, the larger-than-life passions, could never be duplicated elsewhere, and she appeared to know that.

People with DID, acknowledged or not, have usually survived the unsurvivable—whether they remember it or not. They did not fail to thrive and so perish in childhood, as one might reasonably have expected, nor did they commit suicide in adolescence, another bitterly common result. No, they divided themselves, and they survived; and the fact that they survived, and in many cases survived well, probably means that as a group they tend to be, by their original nature, people who have exceptional gifts. Typically they possess intellectual, interpersonal, or creative abilities that might have set them apart from the crowd even if—especially if—their histories had been different. They are superadapters, mind-boggling really. And for some, as for Melissa, an intimate bond with such a person can be an addictive banquet of admiration, fascination, and emotional rushes (in both directions) that is simply not provided by other, more "normal" relationships.

But there is inestimable waste, the waste of a very bright candle at which tragic circumstance has for too long blown a heavy, near-extinguishing mist. The flame may hiss and flash large at times, in impossible displays of protest and vitality that are compelling to witness, but it is always in danger of fading to black.

The talents I refer to are inborn; trauma does not bestow them. Trauma is merely the cruel taskmaster. It rivets our attention, but it is no giver of gifts.

More general than the dissociative identity issue, whether or not psychological pain bestows or perhaps enhances creativity is an old debate. It is the question of, for example, "Would a happy Charles Dickens have written *A Tale of Two Cities*?" In working for many years with a great many traumatized people, artists, musicians, and writers among them, I have answered this question to my own satisfaction, and my answer is this: I do *not* think a happy Charles Dickens would have done less brilliant work, particularly if he were happy because he had recovered from being unhappy. On the contrary, I think that the natural genius of Charles Dickens would have expressed itself even more luminously—and also that the people around him would have led far more comfortable lives.

Happiness is not a mixed blessing.

I tell this opinion to those of my patients who fear they will lose a certain creative edge should they be "cured." One does not lose one's edge. If anything, it becomes a finer blade, and—the best part—one does not have to bleed for it nearly so much. A talented person is not talented because of her or his pain. She or he, like Nathan, is talented despite it. The pain—Nathan's pain—is like a gauzy gray mist that has wrapped itself several times around a priceless clear light.

Nathan's story is especially striking, but it is hardly the only one. On the contrary, examples of unrecognized dissociative identity disorder abound. Individuals who suffer from DID are sometimes in therapy, but much more frequently they are to be found quite outside of any treatment for themselves, as I found Nathan. And each one has a personal history that, like Nathan's, has never been fully investigated.

Thirty-nine-year-old Camisha is from Nigeria, a fascinating place to be from; but she remembers almost none of it. When people ask her, as they often do, about her country of origin, she gives an account that sounds like the "People and Places" section of a travel book. She is articulate, and her descriptions are informative and accurate, but there is nothing personal in them, no emotional attachment, no detailed memories or distinctive examples from her own childhood. When American acquaintances ask her for personal stories, she apologizes and explains that she came to the United States when she was quite young, just eighteen, and has never been back to Nigeria.

"Too young to remember very much, don't you know."

A few of her friends, the ones who are more compassionate and imaginative, make sure not to press her, because they think something terrible must have happened to Camisha in Africa, something unspeakable and exotic, of the type that happens to children only in the Third World. In actuality, however, the terrible thing was, in its basics, all too ordinary and altogether global. Camisha's father and her three older brothers sexually abused her from the age of four until, at the age of twelve, she was able to use her considerable ingenuity and charm to obtain a room at a medical mission. By the time she was eighteen, the intellectually gifted and tenacious Camisha had found passage to New York.

Camisha has no memory of the abuse. She is an American citizen now, a homemaker, living in a small town in Massachusetts, with her husband, a Methodist minister from Brooklyn, and their two teenage children. From her home, she writes and illustrates a winsome series of children's books about a world populated with pastel-colored teddy bears who can talk, and who deliver gentle messages such as, "Love is even better than having lots of toys."

But after all the years, her husband and children have come to accept that, once every few weeks, their usually warmhearted and approachable Camisha will get into her Honda Accord at the beginning of a seemingly random day, and disappear until well after supper, when she will return home and go directly to bed. Her family has learned that it is useless to ask her where she had been on such a day, because the most she will ever say is, "Out. I just went out for a bit."

Also, they learned long ago never to express irritation or anger of any kind toward Camisha, because when they do, her reaction is to become mute and exit to the garden, where for several hours she will sit cross-legged on a favorite flat stone, her back to the house. Slender, straight-backed, and unmoving, at these times she resembles nothing so much as an elegant ebony carving, exquisite but not quite alive. Watching her is almost unbearable, and so is the guilt. Or if the weather is not suitable for the garden, she will simply go to her bedroom and lock the door. Then as a matter of course, and without comment during or after, her husband sleeps on the sofa in the den. In the morning, Camisha is usually her old self again, just as if nothing had happened.

Camisha presents other mysteries as well, and her teenage children are increasingly confused and hurt. Nearly all the time, their beloved mother is sweet and loving toward them, is almost excessively attentive in taking care of their needs—was the favorite neighborhood mom when they were small—and yet, since they have been older, when they try to show her any type of physical affection, give her a hug for instance, she "turns into somebody else," becomes stiff and silent, "sort of like a mannequin in a store." In particular, Camisha's sixteen-year-old daughter has been troubled by this. Always an excellent student, the daughter has recently begun to make below-average grades in school, and to proclaim that she no longer wants to go to college, her single-minded plan since she was old enough to know what college was. She now says she would prefer to stay at home, and perhaps get a job. Strangely, Camisha has said little to oppose this large revision in her talented daughter's ambitions.

The minister-father tries to tell his children that their mother's behavior must have something to do with leftover cultural differences between Nigeria and here.

Eventually, the father will use his church connections to find a clinical social worker who specializes in ethnic family therapy, and Camisha will attend an agreed-upon fifteen sessions with her children and her husband. In the context of such a brief therapy, Camisha's trauma history will not be addressed directly, although the experienced social worker will tacitly assume that she has one, and will therefore refer her to me. But before I even meet her, Camisha will come to understand that certain of her "general anxieties about the world" are inappropriately leaking over, and causing her to sabotage her daughter. In an admirably self-appraising and deliberate fashion, she will begin to encourage the young woman to return to her original plans, to leave home after high school, to become successful and independent. And in the end, with her mother's loving support, the daughter will go away to college in another state. She will major in psychology.

And then there is Charlie, another survivor of severe early abuse, an acquaintance who recently confessed to me that for several years while he was a young man, he would go out on "hero missions" one or two nights every week. A self-nominated vigilante of sorts, Charlie would take his polished blue Belgian-made Browning out of the drawer, holster it under his leather jacket, and in the dead of night, prowl around a certain high-crime district in Baltimore, or sometimes near a particularly isolated late-night market on the outskirts of that city, waiting for the muggers and rapists and holdup artists to appear.

"I couldn't wait. Sometimes if nothing happened at all, I would get so pissed off. I really *needed* that confrontation. Amazing. It's like it happened last night, but at the same time, I can't believe I used to do that stuff. As a matter of fact, I think maybe it wasn't really me, even though I know that sounds crazy as hell."

I asked him to tell me about one of those nights, and he warmed to the task right away.

"Well for instance I'd go to that store, and make like a customer, look around in the corners for a while, away from the front, until some woman came in by herself. Then when she left, I'd pick up a newspaper, throw some money at the register, and follow her, so she never noticed me, just follow her and make sure she got home safe, you know? Most of the time nothing happened. But one night, something did."

"Tell me about it."

But I hardly needed to insist. After just this much, he was already fascinated by his own story, a memory that seemed to come back to him in startling immediacy as he continued to recount it. At fifty-four, Charlie was barrel-chested, and wore his receding steel-gray hair in a little ponytail; but as he lost himself in his story, I could almost have said that his appearance became more youthful. His posture improved, and his gestures were more fluid.

"I got outside, and I watched her cross the street. It was dark, real empty, you know. But after a second I see there's somebody there, some guy standing in a doorway, kind of hidden. Then he comes out to the street, and I see it's some young guy, and I don't like the way he looks, a real punk. And then he starts to follow the girl. She doesn't see him, and he doesn't see me. So I drop the paper and I cross the street, and I, like, start to follow the both of them."

Charlie's speech was becoming rapid and excited, like the narration of an amateur videographer who realizes that he is fortuitously documenting a cataclysm.

"Now he starts to close in on her, and so I put on the speed to catch up to the punk. She never notices anything, just keeps on going. Went home safe, I guess.

"I catch up to the guy—he hasn't heard me yet—and I clap my hand over his shoulder from behind. The guy spins around, but my face is dead calm, man, absolutely dead calm. I'll bet it was spooky. And then—*click!*—this punk's got a switchblade, and he's showing it to me, like sort of telling me I'm dead. His face looks like he's going to kill me. But I just keep on looking calm, you see? Just keep right on looking blank, man, like nothing's there, like maybe I can see right through this guy. And so all of a sudden he starts to look a little worried."

Charlie chuckled, and then altering his voice to sound tough and stupid, began to deliver the punk's side of the dialogue in this little drama:

"'You a cop, man? Hey! I said are you a *cop?* You better say so. You better say so, man.'

"I don't say anything, just keep right on staring. Finally I reach over and just take the blade out of his hand and shut it. He lets me.

"'Hey man, I wasn't doing nothing. I wasn't doing nothing, okay? You gonna bust me for a blade?'

"But all I do is, I look at the knife, and then I flip it over in my hand and look at the other side of it, and then I drop it in my pocket, just like that. Never change my expression. Cold as ice.

"He says, 'Fuck man. You're crazy.'

"I say, 'That's right. I'm crazy. And now I've got your knife, you stupid little slime.'

"He says, 'You ain't no cop,' and then he reaches for me, but I grab his wrist and start to squeeze it real hard, all the time just staring at his eyes with my ice-cold expression. He jerks his arm away, and then he backs off—he was really spooked by then—and he says, 'Okay. Okay, man. Just cool it, okay?'

"And then I smile at him, a big, spooky, I'm-a-crazy-man smile.

"He says, 'Shit. Fucking psycho,' and so then I take a step towards him. He takes two steps back. 'Jesus. I'm gone. I'm gone, man. You stay cool, okay? Stay cool.'

"And then he runs off. Never saw him again."

Charlie gave me an example of his youthful crazy-man smile, and chuckled some more. But then without warning, his face fell, and fifty-four-year-old Charlie looked lost and very sad.

He concluded his tale by saying, "I remember there was this little park near that market, a little park with a kiddy swing set . . . jungle gym . . . whatever. After I'd do something like that thing with the punk chasing the girl, after it was all finished, I'd go over to the park and sit in one of those swings. I'd bend over double, and put my face in my hands, and just swing that way for a while— *creak, creak, creak*—for I don't know how long. In the dark. Just sit there like that. Strange, huh?"

I imagine there was some exaggeration in Charlie's story about the punk, but I imagine also that there was a fair amount of truth in it.

In this and subsequent conversations with Charlie, I discovered that he never killed anyone, and that (miraculously) he was never seriously hurt during any of these episodes. When I asked why he had not pulled his gun, he answered that, once he was on the street, he never took his gun out of its holster. Charlie saw himself not as a killer, but as a protector, an important moral distinction to him (although not an altogether clear one to me), and the Browning he carried was apparently more a symbolic object than a lethal one.

At present, more than thirty years after his "phase" of vigilantism, Charlie owns and manages a booming mail-order vitamin and herbs business, which he created himself ("Rags to riches!"), and he describes himself as a "boring family man" with a wife and three children. In his wildest dreams these days, he cannot imagine involving himself in any kind of violent situation.

"Hell, I don't even like to watch the news on TV."

Charlie is not my therapy patient. In fact, to my knowledge he is nobody's therapy patient. But I suspect that he told me about his past mainly because I am a therapist, because of something about

my demeanor, or perhaps his understanding of what I do profes-
sionally. Although few set out to look for trouble and for people to
protect in quite the way Charlie did, survivors of profound trauma
often do carry weapons, and it is not unusual for a survivor to reveal his or her weapon to someone, particularly to a therapist, or to
some other person who will listen without being judgmental (relatively speaking).

The very first time I saw a weapon in therapy, many years before
I met Charlie, I admit that rather than being frightened, I had to
suppress what would have been a startled laugh. The charming and
prodigiously successful professional woman who, by way of confession, pulled out the shiny switchblade from inside her elegant
calfskin boot (where the knife would probably have been useless
anyway, in the case of a surprise attack upon her) was so patrician
and nonathletic, so carefully made-up and put-together, so gentle,
that the image of her whipping out a deadly blade, and charging in
to go *mano-a-mano* with a burly offender on the street, was unavoidably comical.

I did manage, barely, not to laugh. Thank God.

She had never used the blade, and if she continued her life without actually being assaulted—even in which case she would most
likely not be able to access her inexpertly stowed weapon—she
never would use it. She carried it because of her trauma history,
because carrying the knife, knowing it was there, made her feel
marginally less victimizable, even though the early trauma she had
endured had nothing at all to do with being attacked by a stranger
on the street.

Because of my role as a psychologist, and of people's unpredictable reactions to learning about what I do for a living, I am
sometimes informed, without really wishing to be, about weapons
concealed by individuals not in my care, like Charlie, and sometimes even by absolute strangers. Once, as another illustration, I
was conspiratorially taken aside at a Beacon Hill cocktail party by
a Vietnam-veteran-cum-businessman, who said to me, "I hear you
shrink traumatized people. I'll show you traumatized!"—where-

upon he revealed to me his secret, a hunting knife, carried much more competently than my patient's weapon, not inside his expensive shoe, but on the specially rigged bottom of it. I think he expected me to be shocked, maybe even wanted me to be. But all I felt was sad, for some nineteenish-year-old boy whom I never knew, and who no longer even existed, airlifted away to a jungle by his elders, and left there to deal as best he could with the horrors he would find.

Though I am not usually amused, neither am I appalled or frightened, usually, by the revelations made to me about weapons, and particularly not by those entrusted to me behind the private doors of my session room. Instead, what I experience most often now is the bitter poignancy of the situation, which for me nearly always evokes the picture of a human being starting out innocent and curious in the world, like the little boy visiting the elephant seals at Año Nuevo, only to be ambushed at some point by abominations no innocence could survive. As the years of being a therapist have passed, and with increasing frequency, I find myself having to suppress a rush of tears.

In the aftermath of certain experiences, that one should keep a weapon close at hand is not shocking. It is pragmatic. And a critical benchmark in the therapy of any survivor is reached when he or she is able to feel safe enough in the world to put away the knife or the gun.

Certainly, I have never been threatened—although more than one person has offered to protect me, should I ever need it.

As the years have come and gone, however, what has become frightening to me, terrifying even, is the widespread nature of the phenomenon itself, the variety and the sheer number of people one would not suspect who evidently carry weapons with them wherever they go, most of these people without any memory at all of why they are doing so.

By disclosing my fear, I do not wish to imply that profound early trauma and the dissociative behaviors that result are by themselves the primary cause, or even a major cause, of most varieties of ag-

gression and violence. This is not so. We still know amazingly little about human aggression, though it is a manifestly crucial study
for our society. But we do know enough to recognize that whether
a person, armed or not, will overtly act upon his violent impulses is
determined by a complex and shifting mixture of many factors,
probably including the status of several hormonal and neurological
systems, individual differences in physiological reactivity to stress,
and individual tolerance of, or sensitivity to, disinhibiting substances such as alcohol. Also, there are a number of important
group variables and learning factors, such as differences in economic
pressures, bigotry (versus empathy), cultural attitudes toward violence as a mode of action, and opportunity for observational learning from behavioral models in the media.

Our culture, for instance, would teach us that the effects of even
the most extreme violence last only until the beginning of the next
commercial.

As for the psychiatric causes of lethal violence, these (when they
do play a part, which is far from always) are more likely to be sociopathy (the clinical absence of conscience) or paranoid schizophrenia (fixed persecutory or grandiose delusions—e.g., "I have
been sent by God to eliminate Satan's spawn"—or hallucinations
with persecutory or grandiose content).

But a sense of foreboding comes over me when I think about the
large number of armed trauma survivors who will never be in therapy—some of them quite young, many of them deeply dissociated—precisely because they go about their lives unnoticed *in the
context of* our pressured, media-saturated, violence-exalting society.
Dissociated rage does not know where it came from, or how to direct itself "logically." Such rage, multiplied by the many, and mixed
into the volatile soup of our cultural incitements, is a recipe for
random tragedy. And as we know only too well, random tragedies
we are getting. At moments that catch us most off-guard, and in the
places that seem least likely, the precious and the innocent are lost.

No, even counting in people like Charlie, dissociative reactions
alone are not the primary cause of most kinds of human aggres-

sion; many other factors are more prominent—hormonal and neurological status, disinhibiting substances, social learning, character disorders, fixed delusions. Still, I do get my own special cold chill of suspicion whenever I hear the remark that has now become an American cliché: the former neighbors of the rampage killer declare to the reporter, "He was such a nice, quiet boy. Kept to himself, you know?"

As yet another illustration of dissociative identity disorder, anything but violent, there is Brooke. At twenty-three, tall and broad-shouldered, a committed bodybuilder—and a devoutly feminist law student determined in her chosen work to redress the wrongs of sexism—Brooke speaks to her fiancé in lisping, unnervingly believable baby talk when the two are alone in their Boston apartment. Brooke's friends, who have more than once overheard her sugar-sweet baby talk in the background of a telephone conversation with the fiancé, blame him for this "uncharacteristic" demeanor on her part. They are embarrassed for Brooke, and in discussions with each other, have agreed that, at home, the boyfriend is somehow infantilizing an otherwise independent and dignified young woman.

Though she lived in the medical capital of Boston, Brooke's mother died a horrible death, starting with a diagnosis of advanced breast cancer, when Brooke was six years old. Beginning the week her mother finally died, and continuing until Brooke was fourteen (and starting to menstruate), Brooke's father slept in her bed with her, in the family home. As a young adult, she remembers that her father shared her bed throughout her childhood, but she does not remember anything that happened there. Her close friends who know about this situation think it is strange, but she assures them that nothing untoward occurred.

"It was an awful time. He was lonely. I was lonely. I assume we cuddled, and we slept. And I'm sure that's really all."

From her childhood, Brooke has kept a stuffed koala bear, about eighteen inches tall, frayed and resewn, that she sleeps with even now. When she comes back to the apartment from the gym at night, or from a late lecture on wage discrimination that she was excited to see listed in the *Boston Globe*, more often than not she wraps her long, muscular, adult arms around the bear, and says to her fiancé, "Can Zee-Zee sleep between us tonight? Pweeze, pweeze!"

The boyfriend—who is himself the son of an adored mother who (unbeknownst to him) was abused in childhood—is almost always patient with Brooke's baby talk, and with her request. After all, he loves Brooke. And he knows she will be an incredible lawyer. With her brains and her dedication, Brooke is the sort of person who could really make a difference in the world someday. As for the baby stuff, well, he can live with that, right?

In sharp contrast with Brooke and her fiancé, twenty-seven-year-old Lars is hauled into therapy by his indignant wife, for being a "pathological liar."

While fleshy, sunburned Lars sits silently and stares at his knees, his slender, powder-pale wife points at him and reports to me, "I've finally had all I can take. He lies so much, sometimes I think he doesn't even know how to tell the truth. Lars the Liar, I call him. And he's not just a liar, he's a stupid liar. Sometimes he'll lie about things he did when I was right there myself. I'll ask him why he didn't come home last night, and he'll say he doesn't know what I mean. Or some ridiculous thing, like I'll ask him how come he mowed half the yard and then didn't finish the job, and he'll say he never mowed the yard at all.

"And those are the things that don't matter all that much. The other things, the really bad things—I guess he thinks if he keeps denying it, maybe I'll just let it go. But I can't let it go anymore; it's not right. He hits me sometimes, you know. He's Swedish, for Christ's sake! He's not supposed to hit me! And the next day he'll tell me it never happened. He gets this weird automaton look on his face, and then he'll *swear* it never happened. Makes the hair stand up on the back of my neck. . . ."

This unfortunate young couple may well be ideally (and therefore tragically) matched in their troubles. The husband's especially brittle dissociative identity disorder, which she has construed as his being an inveterate liar—and how is he to argue with that?—effectively distracts the wife from the looming necessity of dealing with her own rageful nature, and could easily do so for a very long time.

Unsurprisingly I suppose, Lars and his wife attended three sessions at my office, and then never came back. During the third session, he had begun, tentatively, to tell me about the various foster parents who had raised him. The next day, she phoned me, politely thanking me for my "help," and despite all my worried protests, said she thought everything would be "much better now." And so I will never know the whole truth about "Lars the Liar"; and neither, I fear, will anyone else.

There is Sarah, a thirty-two-year-old medical assistant who, by her own report and by all appearances, is a well-adjusted, upbeat, "straight arrow," glad to have her good, flexible job, and content as the dedicated mother of a growing young family. And yet in the very back of the guest room closet, neatly concealed behind a stack of blankets that are never used, Sarah keeps an unopened syringe and enough stolen morphine to end her life many times over. These items reside inside a ginger-red cardboard cube tied up with golden twine, that used to house five hundred sheets of perfectly square origami paper.

Once in a while, on a housekeeping binge, she will accidentally come upon her hidden supplies. When this happens, she immediately restashes the box, and leaves the room. Within moments of walking away, she is once again cheerfully amnesic for the fact that she possesses a suicide cache; she could state with wholehearted belief that there is nothing in the closet but blankets.

By chance one especially chilly winter midmorning, Sarah's husband is home alone, with the flu, and while clumsily searching for an extra blanket, pulls out the shiny red box. It tumbles to the floor, where it looks so bright and unusual that he is moved to pull open its golden ties and look inside.

The husband is mystified, and then he is terrified. He phones his wife at work, and she comes home.

Sarah genuinely does not know how or why she has these things, but she realizes they must be hers, because they are obviously from her work. Her husband, who loves her very much but who has a hard time confronting her, suggests she go and have a talk with their rabbi. After two hour-long conversations with Sarah, the rabbi kindly but firmly insists that she see a therapist. He calls me on the spot, to schedule the first appointment for her.

She thinks she feels fine, and she does not want to go to therapy, but she decides she must go anyway, not because she is concerned for her safety (for she still does not understand how this is threatened), but because a powerful set of personal values tells her incontrovertibly that it is wrong to steal things from the medical facility where she works, and where they trust her. If she is stealing drugs from work—and more shameful yet, forgetting that she stole them—then she must do something about it. This is her clear responsibility.

Also, she does not want her poor husband to be so frightened, poor Sam with his milk-bottle glasses and his gentle ways, Sam who loves her even though her hair, the chestnut hair he was so taken with in the beginning, is becoming prematurely white.

Because Sarah's strong sense of responsibility will hold her in therapy, she will eventually remember being sexually abused as a child. And then a lot of things, including the suicide cache, will make more sense, though painfully. In therapy, Sarah will recall her childhood fears that "everything" would somehow be found out, and that she, eight-year-old Sarah, would then be "responsible" for destroying her entire family. And she will find that a dissociated part of her, named "Dossie," believed that "they" (Sarah and "Dossie") should anticipate the horror of such a discovery by being prepared, at a moment's notice, to die.

"Dossie" had worked out that if Sarah were gone, then maybe Sarah's family, everyone she loved, would stand a chance.

Of course, the discovery of incest was never made by Sarah's family. It seldom is made by any family, for people are overwhelmingly motivated not to make it. But "Dossie" remained, and "Dossie" was desperate enough to steal, and hide her plunder.

Happily, loving and responsible Sarah will recover. Given her sense of accountability (both a burden and a blessing), Sam's devotion and encouragement, and an extended therapy that teaches her about trauma and dissociative identity disorder, Sarah will survive the pain of remembering, and be able, ultimately, to integrate herself. And then—with her whole mind—she will denounce the necessity, and even the possibility, of taking her own life.

And there is dainty, small-boned Meng, originally from Cambodia, now a forty-eight-year-old American citizen living in eastern Massachusetts. Meng weighs ninety pounds soaking wet, the youngest and smallest of ten brothers and sisters, and the only member of her Cambodian family to survive the time of the French-Indochinese War.

Meng has finally given in and purchased an air conditioner for her bedroom. Always in the past, she has scoffed at people who needed electric cooling in their homes, proclaiming that no summer heat in this new country of hers, and certainly not in this New England region, could hold a candle to the shimmering green oven of a Cambodian midday. She thinks she must be growing old, for now this trifling American weather is starting to get to her.

As she is driving home with her newly purchased air-conditioning unit, she chances to hear on her car radio the beginning of an especially graphic news report about the fighting far away in Bosnia. Quickly and automatically, she switches the channel to a country music station, and stops listening. But too late. With no awareness of the trip, in less than an instant, Meng makes an involuntary mental journey all the way from where she is in Massachusetts to Yugoslavia, and from Yugoslavia across the world to the lush Mekong River basin, where she becomes a different person—the person who relies on herself alone, the one who survives.

Back at the store, two large, muscular people struggled to put Meng's air conditioner box into the trunk of the old Cadillac. But when diminutive Meng arrives home, just as the country music station is going to commercial, she hoists the unit out of the trunk, carries it into her house, and single-handedly installs it in an upstairs window.

The next morning, when her six-foot, thoroughly American son happens to see it, and to ask her how on earth it got there, she honestly does not know, nor can she figure out why she is suddenly so bruised.

And then there is Mason. Mason's childhood was spent with his sadistically violent alcoholic father, his "utterly annihilated" mother, and his older brother, in a place Mason usually refers to now as "Nowhere-at-all, South Dakota." His father made enough money for liquor and food, in that order, as a last-stop, self-proclaimed mechanic who patched together broken farm machinery, small trucks, and the occasional automobile.

When Mason's brother was fifteen, he ran away from home, and Mason, eleven at the time, never saw him again. Mason's mother died (of heart failure, said the county coroner) when he was seventeen. Mason had felt he should not abandon his mother, but after she died, he himself got away from "home" by going to Vietnam, when he was eighteen, and so out of that frying pan into the fire.

Today Mason, with wild gray hair and a great forest of a beard, is fifty years old, and a university professor living and working in London. He teaches American history there, a subject in which he earned a Ph.D., after the war. ("Uncle Sam bought it for me," he says.) He sometimes impresses his students in London with the vastness of his childhood isolation by telling them, in his best American twang, that even these days a person would have to drive five hours from "Nowhere-at-all, South Dakota," just to get to the vicinity of a small airport. Most of the young people are incredulous at this. And privately, he congratulates himself that, at least within the English-speaking world, Goodge Street is about as far away, geographically and culturally, as one could possibly get from South Dakota. Nothing in London looks like, feels like, or even smells like, anything at all from his childhood.

Mason is a good man, with a good heart. Nine years ago, he married a gentle, intelligent Englishwoman, younger than he, and somewhat late in his life, started a family with her in what he gratefully saw as his new home. Their two young children, a boy and a girl, seem to bring him unending delight, and friends and colleagues remark that apparently Mason was born to be a father.

He is a good teacher as well. He infuses his lectures with the compassionate, if somewhat drifty, politics of American 1960s liberalism, and he is (ironically) very effective at imparting George Santayana's old, wise warning that "those who cannot remember the past are condemned to repeat it." Also, barbarities in Vietnam, following on the heels of his own father's vicious behavior, taught him well that might is not always right, by any means. He instructs his students to be watchful, and to question authority figures, beginning with him, if they wish.

From time to time, Mason will congenially roll up his left sleeve to show his students the tattoo on his forearm that he acquired as a much younger man, a small peace sign etched in interlocking blue and yellow flowers.

But sometimes Mason is a different person altogether. Occasionally, and for no obvious reason, he becomes an unreasoning Victorian-style tyrant in his home, seething with inexplicable anger at his young children, and icily sending them away to bed at six in the evening. Mason's wife, who after nine years of marriage is secretly somewhat afraid of Mason, "walks on eggshells" around him, in a vain attempt to prevent his "getting into a mood." She feels a constant, sickening dread of these "moods" in her "usually quite marvelous" husband, because they sometimes develop into non-negotiable refusals to speak at all, to her or to her children. These merciless silences can last for days, or even longer. Once Mason was mute for two entire weeks. And then one Sunday morning, he simply woke up as himself again, as if nothing unusual had happened.

Mason's wife, exhausted, pretended the same.

Such a list of unrecognized DID sufferers could go on almost indefinitely, and a few readers may already be thinking that there are some uncannily familiar descriptions here. In any event, reminiscent of personal acquaintances or not, Nathan and the others are far from otherworldly. On the contrary, in surprisingly large numbers, they populate our own, quite ordinary, world.

What are they like, these switchers? Publicly, they can give the appearance of greater-than-normal adaptability, but when one knows them up close, they can be brittle people, unstable, hard to count on. Often, one hears complaints from family members, like Mason's wife, that one must walk on eggshells around them. By definition, they are changeable, often disturbingly so; there is a recognized personality, considered by others to be the "normal" one, but this personality sometimes switches to one or more alternate emotional and behavioral patterns, deemed (by others) to be completely "out of character," and therefore objectionable or even unbearable.

Some people with dissociative identity disorder switch frequently, perhaps every week or even every day, and others switch only occasionally. To confuse the picture still more, some individuals, like Charlie, may endure a phase of frequent switching, followed by years of not switching at all. Like Charlie, they may have personal histories that sound impossibly "out of character." A person affected in this way may possess a strange, foreign-feeling memory of having been "someone else," recollections from the life of a radical, encapsulated self that seemingly got left behind.

Having been switched to, an alternate personality does not respond to cajoling from other people, to outcry, or even to the most desperate pleas for a return to "normal." (In other words, when someone has lost his observing ego, you cannot tell him much.) Unlike the phenomenon of "moodiness," which may very well accommodate the needs of other people, or react to a favorable turn of events, a dissociative identity is impermeable. Once in place, it has a life of its own, in the most fascinating and frustrating sense of that phrase. And after an unpredictable interval of time, independently of anyone else's efforts, or of changes in circumstance, it seems to disappear on its own.

Often there can be a crazy-making holographic effect for a life partner, a child, or a close friend: the switcher is loving/vicious/loving/vicious, or wise/infantile/wise/infantile, or noble/corrupt/noble/corrupt. This fluttering perception never resolves; the question, "What is this person really like?" is never conclusively answered. And in the end, a switcher whom one loves dearly can seem to be simultaneously one's best friend, and in some peculiar, ineffable way, one's most terrible enemy.

Also, to be the intimate of a switcher is to live alongside someone with highly inconsistent powers of memory, and this feature of the experience may be even more distressing for the unsuspecting companion than is the individual's changeability itself. The switcher's "normal" capacity to remember even the smallest details of recent events may seem extraordinary, or hypervigilant. But sometimes, strangely, he may relate the same story to the same person more than once, seemingly unaware that he has passed this information before. Or sometimes he may forget that the person he is addressing was the one who told him the story in the first place. Or sometimes he may forget that he has done a task, and set about to do it again.

Of course, we all tend to forgive a certain amount of forgetfulness in another person. When the incident is not significant, we

say to ourselves that the one who does not remember was distracted, or stressed. But when a switcher states that he has no
memory whatsoever of an intensely meaningful event that happened, say, yesterday afternoon, another person who was involved
in the event is bound to become spooked or, more probably, en-
raged. A screaming argument is quite likely to ensue.

Switchers tend to make other people very angry.

And making their companions angry is but one of the ways in
which people with DID can appear to be working at cross-
purposes with themselves. Like Nathan, who missed out on an
elaborate gala of his own creation, and who tormented a wife for
whom he wished only happiness, switchers can seem mystifyingly
intent upon punching ever-enlarging holes in their own lives. Since
people in relationships with the switcher virtually never recognize
his disorder, they formulate their own explanations for his
maddening behaviors (self-confident nonconformity, irrational
jealousy, pathological lying, and so forth), but these entirely reasonable portrayals often have little or nothing to do with what is
really happening.

And so, most switchers are interpersonally brittle, changeable,
impervious to input, intermittently amnesic, and generally crazy-
making. Also, most are walking, talking "projective devices," a
term used by psychologists to describe things (for example, ink-
blots) that by virtue of the extremely ambiguous picture they
present, invite us to project our own conflicts and ideas upon them.
We see what we want to see, or what we *need* to see, in people who
are ambiguous. Perhaps this is another reason why friends and
lovers stay in relationships with such people: at least some of the
time, we can imagine them to be anyone we desire.

These are the features of most switchers. Interestingly, two features that do *not* characterize most switchers are 1) conspicuous
naming of alter personalities, and 2) highly dramatic changes in
behavioral markers such as speech pattern, vocal type, facial expression, and postural habit. The small percentage of switchers
who do, like my patient Garrett, overtly name their alters, and un-

dergo breathtaking changes in voice and physical appearance, constitute only a distinctive minority within a much larger group.

We picture a well-groomed and appealing Dr. Jekyll, and a hunched and craggy Mr. Hyde. And we have seen the dramatic outward transformations in *The Three Faces of Eve*, for which, in 1957, Joanne Woodward won the Academy Award for Best Actress. And this, even now, is what we expect of dissociative identity disorder. We expect a refined Dr. Jekyll and a snarling Mr. Hyde. We expect riotously diverse and immediately recognizable characters, such as those in Flora Rheta Schreiber's *Sybil*, and the 1976 film version. But the simple fact is that most individuals, dissociative or not, are incapable of visually and dramatically revealing their internal experience. Most of us are inadequate actors, and our internal states—whether these be complex dissociated alters or simple, nondissociated feelings—are almost never conveyed with great clarity to other people.

Sarah Bernhardt, had she been afflicted with DID, would have been florid, frightening, brilliant when she switched. Her ego states would have been theatrically portrayed and arrestingly distinct. She would have *become* them, on the outside as well as on the inside. But few people have the abilities of a Sarah Bernhardt or a Joanne Woodward, to be used either voluntarily or involuntarily. Most of us, if we switched, would *look* much like we usually do, and no one at all would say "Wow!" Imagine William Hurt or Sir Anthony Hopkins or the late Andy Kaufman trying to project an alternate personality to people looking on from the outside. And now imagine your next-door neighbor—or perhaps yourself—endeavoring to do the same thing.

No, most people do not, cannot effectively portray their inner lives to the world. Nathan the doctor sometimes became "nuclearblast" rageful, according to his wife, Melissa, but he never defined the situation fully for her by distorting his face and body into that of Stevenson's Mr. Hyde. Camisha assumed the demeanor of a statue, but she certainly did not convert and morph and transmogrify like Garrett, or Sybil Isabel Dorsett in *Sybil*, or Chris Costner Sizemore as depicted in *The Three Faces of Eve*. The highly dissociative Lars—well, he just seemed like a garden-variety liar. And congenial Mason became impenetrably silent for days on end, but he always *looked like* Mason.

The spellbinding attribute of visible metamorphosis—the feature that has so preoccupied both popular and scientific attention where the "rare disease" of dissociative identity disorder is concerned—is the product of something more complex than DID alone. The tendency to metamorphose outwardly is perhaps the interaction of DID with certain other characteristics. In the absence of DID, some of these other predispositions, such as greater-than-average self-hypnotic ability (focused imagination), remarkable empathic perception (understanding what emotions feel like and look like), and a superior aptitude for mimicry and impersonation, would probably be referred to as natural gifts. To be specific, they are endowments that in other circumstances might lead the individual to be an amateur method actor, or even a professional one.

By chance, these "acting" gifts may occasionally be found in someone who has DID *as well*, and in tandem with the various ego states, may result in the dramatic transformations popularly ascribed to "multiple personality disorder." In other words, if a person with DID happens to be especially brilliant at projecting her internal experience to the outside, then her dissociated ego states—which are most definitely a part of her internal experience—will tend to be brilliantly portrayed, automatically and unconsciously. But since most people with DID have no more acting ability than any of the rest of us, most dissociative episodes are far from dazzling to an outside observer.

For example, Garrett's identity disorder was a painfully involuntary part of his real life, not in his direct control; but if he could have voluntarily done the same thing in a stage production, he would have received a standing ovation. Very few people with dissociative identity disorder, very few people of any kind, are so talented. Most—Nathan, Camisha, Sarah, Mason, and all the many unrecognized others—possess no rare and stunning theatrical powers to be unconsciously applied to their dissociated ego states. Their transformations do not amaze, beguile, or petrify us. From a little distance, they look almost like ordinary people, and in a sense, they are.

PART FOUR

SANITY

CHAPTER EIGHT

Why Parker Was Parker

The human soul is very much older than the human mind.

—Konrad Lorenz

The dissociative nature of our consciousness can create show-stopping disruptions in our personal relationships, in our parenting efforts, and even in our capacity to function well as a society. As illustrations of the impact upon lives and upon the community, the internationally respected expert on traumatic stress, Bessel A. van der Kolk, has reported cases in which forgotten traumatic experiences were reenacted in complex and extraordinary ways. In 1987, van der Kolk published the study of a woman, referred to as Melody D., who was completely amnesic for having survived the 1942 Coconut Grove nightclub fire in Boston, in which 492 people perished. Though she had lost all memory of the tragedy, she would reenact her experience on its anniversary. For example, Melody would suddenly begin to ask her fellow, presumably mystified, hospital patients, "How many women did you save from the fire? How many did you carry out?" This study of

Melody D. was followed, in 1989, by the account of a Vietnam vet-
. eran who effectively set up police to engage in a gun battle with
him precisely on the anniversary of his friend's death in Vietnam,
even though the veteran possessed no conscious memory of the
original violent event.

But one does not really have to look to professional journals to
find important instances of interpersonal and social disruption
caused by dissociative behavior, especially switching. The complex
and the extraordinary are in the medical literature. But the simple
and the ordinary, the repeated patterns that affect us all, can be
found anywhere.

Perhaps the most obvious example is the devastation that occurs
in a relationship when one or both members of a couple are unrecognized switchers. Because an active dissociated ego state is change-
less and seamless, it cannot be related to and communicated with,
at least not in the same ways that one member of a couple has
learned to use customarily with the other. As a result, the non-
switcher who is trying to communicate will immediately feel frustrated, anxious, or angry, and may ultimately come to feel lonely,
incompetent, and depressed. For the switcher himself, the repeated psychological isolation from the other person, which by
definition occurs when the switcher is frightened or hurt, will serve
to deprive him of almost all emotional support. In the long run,
when he is functioning as a dissociated ego state, he is likely to be
either angrily ranted at by the other person, or stonily ignored.

Also, even beyond the inaccessibility of emotional support, at
these times a switcher is prevented from taking in another person's
emotional responses as useful *information* about relationships. This
situation is especially tragic for someone who may already be suffering from trauma-related *alexithymia* (loss of the ability to recognize specific emotions of one's own, that would otherwise serve as
judicious guides for responding to other people). The alexithymic
individual cannot identify his own feelings, or convey them in
words. Instead, he may express uncomfortable emotional states as
aggressive acts against himself or others, or as recurring psychoso-

matic symptoms that he cannot perceive as emotionally determined. A dissociative identity disorder into the bargain makes it all
but impossible for the emotionally illiterate person to modify his
ignorance secondarily, by receiving the positive emotional lessons
that might have been provided by nondisrupted contact with loved
ones and companions.

"When he gets like that and I try to get close, he's like a snarling
wolf guarding his cave," grieves one spouse. "It's so crazy. I mean,
I'm about the least threatening creature I can imagine."

But what she really cannot even imagine are the savage threats
that did exist in his childhood, from which he needed to protect a
small and unimaginably vulnerable lair, and which forced him, in
the interest of survival, to keep his instinctive emotional reactions
at a distance. At the time, a lot of snarling probably helped. But
now that he is older, it only insures that he will remain a lonely
man, perhaps for the rest of his life.

Dissociative identity disorder uses an antique shovel to widen an
intensely frustrating chasm that keeps opening and closing, reap-
pearing and disappearing, between the unacknowledged switcher
and his mate, and even his own creative potential. Oblivious to
everything but the unspeakable past, the disorder is not moved by
aching disconnections that may last a lifetime, or by the irrecover-
able waste of joy, talent, and human comfort.

Less obvious than the couple disruptions, but perhaps even
more devastating, are the effects upon a child of having a parent
who is a switcher. From a parent's alter ego that is hostile, or hostile-
paranoid, a child, even one who is quite beloved by the switcher,
may derive a lifelong image of himself as suspect, unworthy, bad.
Living with a parent's dissociated ego state that is immature, helpless, naive, even a very young child may attempt to trade roles with
the parent, and begin to view herself as the perennial caregiver.

Mason, the liberal university professor who sometimes switches
to an autocratic tyrant at home, may well end up with grown children who, though they are not switchers, do experience themselves
as contemptible, and therefore cringe and submit before precisely

those guises of authority the professor himself most despises. Brooke, the conscientious feminist law student who switches at times to an innocent little-girl personality may someday raise a daughter who, having begun as a preschooler to take care of her lawyer-mother when she switched, fully assumes the negative female stereotype of sacrificing all her needs to others, whether or not they mistreat her. The nature of long-term self-defeat in DID is often just this ironic.

Most grievous of all—a dissociated ego state who is a child molester may perpetuate child abuse across yet another generation, without any apparent knowledge that he or she is doing so.

I came face-to-face with this last chilling possibility some years ago, in the course of treating a young man who suffered from chronic anxiety and addiction to Valium. When he was a child, the patient had been sexually abused by his father's older sister, and while he was in treatment with me, out of the clear blue sky he received a nine-page letter from this aunt, confessing to and apologizing for the very abuse he had been discussing in our sessions. Both the patient and I were astounded by the letter; child abusers seldom admit their acts, and for her to do so spontaneously in this way was something on the order of a miracle. After getting the apology, the patient wanted his aunt to attend one of his therapy sessions, so that he could discuss the past with her, and also tell her, in person, what her abusive behavior had cost him psychologically. He and I were both stunned again when she unhesitatingly agreed to a three-way meeting at my office. On the telephone, she told him, quite composedly, that she loved him, and would "naturally" do anything she could to help him.

The patient was strongly affected by this, because he felt that, at twenty-four years old, he still loved her, too, despite the fact that she had hurt him, and even though he had not seen her at all since he was eighteen. His feelings were understandable. She had been one of his most important caregivers when he was a small boy, and he could recount to me instances of her devotion, an affection sickeningly distorted and stained by abuse. He believed that if, in his presence, she could express remorse, then he could forgive her, and thereby be several steps closer to his recovery. He even expressed a wish that she might seek out a therapist for herself. I had my doubts, not about his capacities, but about hers.

I remember that before the scheduled time of the meeting, I worried a little obsessively about how I would go about shaking the hand of this confessed child molester when she arrived. Practitioner of a compassionate profession or not, I felt that I should fix her with an accusatory glare, rather than simply greet her as if she were anybody else. It afforded me some guilty relief to reflect that often when two women meet, they do not shake hands anyway.

The aunt, looking just exactly like anybody else, arrived at my office right on time, said a warm hello to her nephew, and in a most mannerly fashion, held out a hand for me to shake. I shook it, and we all sat down.

For the first three or four minutes, acting as my patient's advocate, I explained what I thought he wanted to get out of the meeting, which was, in short, an elucidation of past events, and an in-person resolution. Watching him with concern, I saw that, though nervous, he was thoughtfully prepared for this strange occasion; he radiated a certain quiet dignity, and was wearing his "job interview wing tips," freshly shined. Also, and this to my alarm, his boyish face betrayed much more hope for the outcome than he had admitted to me in previous sessions. For her part, the aunt was a stylish, kinetic woman in her mid-fifties, with shoulder-length shiny black hair, who kept changing her position to look curiously around my office, but who certainly did not seem distressed in any way. The surprising thought occurred to me that, of the three of us there, I was the one with the most trepidation.

Then I turned to the aunt, who spoke easily and articulately. She said that she had come to the meeting because she loved her nephew deeply, that she felt like a second mother, and wanted to end their estrangement, if possible. When he had phoned her about coming to his therapy, she had viewed the overture from him as a prayed-for opportunity. I looked at my patient again. His eyes were moist, and he was obviously moved. I asked him whether he had anything to say at that point, and he answered that he had brought the letter, and would like to give it to her now, so that she could review it, and then maybe we could all talk. I nodded, and he handed her the thick envelope.

Without comment, she opened it and read, closely, for nearly ten minutes. After about five, my patient, who had not anticipated such a painstaking review, sighed shakily, and said that he needed to go and get some water. In his absence, I continued to watch the aunt read, her dark eyebrows pinched in effortful concentration, her eyes dry. She held the papers first in her right hand, then in her left, moved in her chair, and crossed and recrossed her legs several times. The nephew came back into the room just as she reached the last page. She refolded the letter, placed it in the envelope, and returned it to him.

"This is really awful," she said. "Why did you show it to me?"

"I thought we could discuss it here," he answered, looking across at her expectantly. "I guess . . . I guess first of all I'd like to find out why you chose now to write it. I mean, why you waited so long."

"Write it? I don't understand. I didn't write that letter."

There followed a moment of silence, during which the nephew—and I—were too amazed to speak. Then, shaking his head as if to clear some misunderstanding, he said, "What do you mean?"

"I mean just what I said. I didn't write that letter."

"Of course you wrote the letter. You sent it to me. You signed it. Look here."

He took the letter out of the envelope again, and held up the last page for her to see.

In the ensuing five minutes, an argument took place, tentative at first, and then painfully emotional on my patient's part, that threatened to deteriorate into his fairly pleading with the woman before him to admit that she had written the letter now in his lap. I could readily understand his frantic attempts, since I myself felt that I had just stumbled into a reality-crumpling scene from some absurdist play. And for him, her mind-boggling behavior was dealing the final deathblow to an important childhood relationship, and the fragile wishes and hopes still linked to the past.

But his aunt continued resolutely, almost patiently, to insist that she had not written the letter. When asked why she thought her nephew had refused to see her for the past six years—since she did not believe for one moment that she had ever perpetrated child abuse—her answer was that she assumed she had said or done something to make him angry, but for the life of her, she did not know what. In fact, she said, she had come to the meeting to ask him what it was, and maybe even get things straightened out.

My patient was becoming more and more desperate, clearly to no avail, and I decided to conclude the meeting early by dismissing the aunt. At the door, as she left us, she turned back briefly and once again told her nephew that she loved him and missed him, and wished that there were some way to end the bad feelings between them. She appeared to be entirely sincere. She even offered to come back for another meeting, if he thought it would help. She had, she said gently, taken no offense at all from his accusations.

She was gone less than half an hour after she had arrived, but in that short time had done enough harm to consume the rest of that session, and many sessions to come, in my doing extensive damage control with her shaken nephew. Fortunately, this particular individual, young as he was, possessed the wisdom to know that—regardless of anything his aunt had ever done to him, or said, or believed—he alone was responsible for his own life and actions. This philosophy mercifully tended to take the focus off his aunt, who was apparently quite lost, to him and to herself. His personal conviction gave him dignity, and in the end, the strength to complete his recovery despite her.

She was more than one woman, his aunt, and her dissociative identity disorder sketched the design for a compartmentalized life during which she maimed a child she loved, and deprived herself of his companionship for all time. It even scratched out her attempts to make amends.

To switch and commit child abuse, and then not to remember. A more horrifying destiny is difficult to imagine. But, the heart-stopping corollary of this circumstance is that conceivably there are other, even more far-reaching possibilities. For example, what if a luminary or a leader—someone in a position of power not in the context of one family only, but in the context of a whole community, or a trusted institution, or a nation—were to be, in addition, a switcher? The potential for the abuse and subversion of an entire society is stupefying.

And so, in our dealings with each other—personal, parental, and political—are we consistent in anything? What organizes our responses, our choices? If not personality, which will fragment unpredictably under enough stress, then what is the unifying feature of a human being (besides, of course, the singularity of the biological unit itself)? Is there such a feature at all? Is there an essential piece in each of us that reviles what it reviles, and cherishes what it cherishes, and never the twain shall meet?

Where is the soul?

One might easily imagine that dissociative identity disorder—given its antithetical combinations of violent personalities, and meek personalities, and promiscuous personalties, and puritanical personalities, and so forth—would, overall, yield a kind of net-neutral in terms of the individual's value system or moral character. But I can tell you that this is not the case. I have known switchers who were narcissists across the board, and some who were frightening sociopaths, and still others who, when appraised across all their personalities, were self-effacing heroes, radiantly moral and conscientious almost to a fault. Far from nullifying the concept of soul, as some fear it will, familiarity with dissociative identity disorder causes me, even with my scientific pretensions, to feel significantly more inclined toward the idea. Something is there—something energetic enough to shine through all the neurological compartmentalization and obfuscation of our selves, and to illuminate and guide, for better or for worse, the multiform unit we think of as "person."

The most dazzling manifestation of this guiding entity that I have witnessed occurred in one of the most severe cases of DID that has ever come to my attention. Parker's dissociative disorder was so profound that she might switch several times a day, from a seething, self-loathing isolate, to a sweet, needy "five-year-old girl," to a brazen seductress, to the shy, likable "main" personality of the twenty-two-year-old woman she was, and dizzyingly back again. But every single one of her alters took tender, responsible care of her bright-eyed, fearless two-year-old daughter. Parker's own early childhood, which had been spent in a remote shanty in the Appalachian Mountains, had been fantastically nightmarish, and had predictably taken its toll. But nothing was going to happen to Parker's little daughter, not if Parker could prevent it.

When Parker was Parker, she was a gifted mother, playful, gentle, an inspiration to watch as she delighted in her two-year-old child. And I am sure she would have been the very soul of maternal ferocity, had anything threatened.

Then there were the alters.

One of these, the isolate, was self-destructive. She would steal razor blades, and make gory cuts into the skin of her own upper arms and the flesh of her belly, and then usually take herself to an emergency room. Each time the self-loathing alter was about to commit such an atrocity against herself, she would make sure that the two-year-old daughter was safely in the care of another person she could count on, far away from the to-be bloody scene. She would give reassuring excuses for her absences to the baby-sitter, and had created elaborate safeguards against the child's ever catching sight of the cutting, the wounds, or even the resulting scars.

The temptress personality gave the child secret little song-lessons in ladylike good manners—please and thank you—and scrupulously concealed, from any men who might be around, the fact that she had a young daughter at all.

When Parker switched to a "five-year-old girl," it was at once unsettling and poignant to see her toddling along, sucking her left thumb, and protectively enfolding with her right hand the tiny fist of an actual two-year-old child, a real toddler who was, at that moment, a mere three cognitive years younger than her mother. At two, Parker's daughter did not suck her own thumb. She appeared to feel entirely secure.

I do not mean to imply that the daughter was growing up in good circumstances. Inevitably, her sense of safety in the world would be seriously undermined by the outrageous inconsistencies in her mother's identity. I do mean to say that the daughter was immeasurably better off than if Parker's various ego states had not been united by maternal love and a total acceptance of accountability. And I mean to communicate my sense of wonder regarding Parker herself. Much of the time, this turbulently dissociative woman could not remember her own legal name; but she could always remember what was most important in her life. Somehow, her sense of responsibility to her child—motherhood's strength of meaning—was superordinate to (or perhaps more fundamental than) her voracious identity disorder.

Countless writers, philosophers, and yes, even scientists, have remarked upon the importance of meaning—relational, moral, spiritual, aesthetic—in the organization of the human mind. Nowhere is the organizing capacity of meaning so observable as in individuals where other, more traditionally assessed functions of mind have been compromised or lost through physical injury or disease. Professor of Clinical Neurology at Albert Einstein College of Medicine, Oliver Sacks—the mesmerizing "anthropologist of the mind"—writing of a profoundly incapacitated Korsakoff's syndrome patient he calls Jimmie G., is, as usual, particularly eloquent in addressing this subject.

Korsakoff's, associated with the thiamine deficiency sometimes seen in long-term alcohol abuse, is a syndrome of amnesia, among other debilities, caused by lesions of the mammillary bodies and of other parts of the brain and brainstem. The organically mediated amnesia of demented and helpless Jimmie G. was so extensive that he had completely forgotten most of the past, and was unable to remember, for longer than a few seconds, anything new presented to him. He was "isolated in a single moment of being, with a moat or lacuna of forgetting all round him." However, to his surprise, Sacks realized that if Jimmie G. were listening to music, or especially if he were taking part in Mass at the chapel in the Home for the Aged where he lived, he could concentrate steadily, and participate fully in the experience. There was "no Korsakoff's then . . . for he was . . . absorbed in an act, an act of his whole being, which carried feeling and meaning in an organic continuity and unity."

Where dissociative identity disorder is concerned, too, a system of meaning—an aesthetic system, or a spiritual one, or a person-oriented and moral one such as Parker's—may succeed in unifying a "whole being" whom a fractured personality system is unable to unify. Of course, when we apply value judgments, as we invariably do, any particular system of meaning may be viewed by us as either positive or negative, helpful or harmful, or somewhere in between. For example, a meaning structure that says, "I love my child, and she is my first responsibility," will probably be seen as positive, while a scheme that dictates, "Me first, at all costs," will be perceived as generally negative. But both of these value/meaning systems, regardless of valence, would appear to be cogent organizers of the mind, even a mind ravaged by psychological trauma.

Given the work I do, I naturally ponder whether there are any organizing systems of meaning and value—"good" ones or "bad" ones—that correlate with successful recovery from dissociative disorders, or any that militate against such an outcome. Are there souls, so to speak, for whom the prognosis is better than for others? And when I consider all my patients, over all the years, the answer is yes: there is in fact an astonishingly robust correlation between an individual's successful recovery on the one hand, and on the other hand, a person's preexisting conviction that she and she alone is *responsible* for something. This something could be an endeavor or a specific person, or is quite likely to be the conduct of her life in general. People who are compelled and organized by a sense of responsibility for their actions tend to recover.

And conversely, sadly, people whose directive meaning systems do not include such a conviction tend not to recover, tend to remain dissociatively fragmented and lost.

This distinction is other than that of perceived locus of control—Who has the power, I or the universe?—which is an understandably double-edged issue for nearly all survivors of trauma. Rather, the difference is that of tenaciously assuming personal responsibility for one's own actions, and therefore taking on personal risk, versus placing the highest valuation upon personal safety, both physical and emotional, which often precludes the acknowledgment of responsibility. (If I acknowledge responsibility toward my child—or my friend or my ideas or my community—then I may be compelled to stick my neck out. I may have to do, or feel, something that will make me more vulnerable.) Here, the psychology of trauma comes full circle, in that the original function of dissociation is to buffer and protect; and so by rights, patients who value self-protection above all else should be candidates for treatment failure, even though they may experience, in addition, an ambivalent wish to be rid of their devitalizing dissociative reactions.

A self-protective system of mind may express itself behaviorally in many ways. Three of the most common ways can be characterized as action-avoidant dependency upon another person or upon a confining set of rules, a preoccupation with reassigning blame, and actions and complaints that indicate a lack of perspective on one's own problems relative to the problems of others. In dissociative identity disorder, such behaviors—just like their "responsible" opposites in a very different "soul"—may be observed, along with some distracting variations in style, across all of the various personalities.

The third behavioral expression of a self-protective soul—acting upon a lack of perspective on one's own problems relative to those of others—is reflected in our society at large by the popular phenomenon of victim identification. Victim identification presupposes the belief that there is a finite group of victims within the larger population, and that one is either a member of this group or not. Membership is (paradoxically) attractive because it affords, first and foremost, a sense of belonging, and after that, all the special status, sympathy, and considerations typically given to those who have been preyed upon and hurt. Also, as an identity, as something *to be*, it may fill up the terrifying sense of emptiness that often follows trauma.

Unfortunately, forever holding on to an identity as victim bodes ill for the person's recovery from that very trauma. Holding fast to this way of seeing oneself and the world can keep an individual endlessly beguiled by his own misery. Also, victim identification blinds its subscribers to the leveling fact that we have all—yes, granted, some more so than others—but we have *all* been hurt at one time or another. We are in this together: patients, non-patients, therapists, everyone.

For these reasons, it is crucial that a fine balance be struck by therapists, and by anyone wishing to help those with DID, or any other dissociative disorder—in the session room, in the home, in survivors groups, and even in the newly developed context of mental health Web sites and chat rooms. A survivor of trauma is a victim, certainly; but "victim" does not comprise the totality of her, or anyone else's, identity. Helpers must support the healing process in both of its phases: the survivor must endure the discovery that she is a victim, and then she must take responsibility for being that no longer. Both parts are equally important, and in neither phase can self-protection be the primary goal. Enabling someone's long-term identity as a victim robs her of an important human right, that of being responsible for her own life.

Also, whether or not a particular person is willing, after a time, to relinquish the status of victim is important information for a helper, because it tends to predict who will and who will not recover. In this regard, I sometimes gently point out to a patient that if she will reflect for a moment, she will probably realize that extreme victim identification and self-pity were, truth to tell, prominent characteristics of her *abuser*. And is this really how she wants to live her whole life, too?

The prognostic information provided by the relative strength of responsibility and self-protection in organizing the mind would lead one to predict, for example, that my patient Garrett, even with all his dramatic, named alters, will recover—and that my other patient's letter-writing aunt will never do so. This is my best guess, even though the aunt's dissociative identity disorder itself is presumably far less spectacular than Garrett's.

In many ways, close study of dissociative behavior supports an old truth, that we cannot simultaneously protect ourselves and experience life fully. These two desires preclude each other proportionately. To the extent that we try to protect ourselves, we cannot truly live; and to the extent that we truly live, we cannot place our highest value upon protecting ourselves. This lesson is not new, but it is interesting that the theme reiterates itself right down to our neurological blueprints. Maybe there is no salvation for any of us outside of the meaning system provided by personal responsibility, despite all the daunting risks. Perhaps this is why we so doggedly look for examples of accountability in our role models, our parents, our leaders.

Dissociative identity disorder—and all of the even more subtle dissociative reactions—rob us of our present reality, and create disruptions in our interpersonal lives, sometimes catastrophic ones. And ultimately, our dissociative behavior causes us, in an ironic vicious circle, to be more at risk, to be more vulnerable to the potential global traumas that threaten the life of our species as a whole. For any of us, switchers or not, to discuss crises such as stockpiled weapons of mass destruction, organized genocide, environmental atrophy, and pandemic starvation is so frightening that we dissociate from our true emotions within seconds, and our conversations are over-intellectualized and motivationally bereft. We do not take effective action; we take a mental exit.

Will this unhinged awareness be with us to some bitter end, or can we regain our sanity? Can we recapture our ongoing reality, reenter the present moment, stay connected with our selves and with our lovers, our friends, our children—our planet? How do we recognize and take responsibility for our dissociative behavior, and for helping the other adults in our lives?

If you are living with a switcher, your main concern will naturally be with how to change him, how to make him into a non-switcher, how to transform him into his "real" self. The truth is that for any human being to change significantly is a massive undertaking. The odds are lined up against success, and there are no odds whatsoever if the person himself is not interested in being different, is not sincerely inclined, for his own crystal-clear reasons, to take on the stupendous project of changing himself.

Still, some information may be helpful.

Occasionally, a person may consider therapy if he is sympathetically confronted, by another person, with the extent of his own memory disturbance. For a life partner or a close friend to point out to the switcher that he loses time, that he apparently has no memory for meaningful things he has recently said and done, may be motivating. Most people want to be in control of themselves, as a high priority, and to have no recall for consequential blocks of time is a sign that one is embarrassingly, maybe even perilously, out of control. When someone else notices, always remarks, and does not excuse such incidents as examples of normal forgetting, an individual is sometimes propelled toward help, if only for his recurrent control-robbing amnesia.

This life partner or this friend must not attempt to take charge of the switcher's life; the switcher, like anyone else, must ultimately make his own decisions. Overall, in fact, not trying to take charge of the switcher's condition is the most important suggestion I can provide to anyone living with such a person. When he switches, and you feel you cannot reach him—because he is someone you hardly even recognize—remember always that his condition of mind was established before you met him, probably long before, and is entirely outside your sphere of direct influence. Of course, accepting this is both a relief and a heartache.

Take care of yourself. If someone switches to a rageful, violent personality, get away, leave. Remaining there will change nothing, will not help you or the switcher, and may well result in your being injured. Staying is precisely as risky as proximity to any other rageful, violent person.

If you are absolutely certain that an alter is not frightening, and is being merely unresponsive and frustrating, know that you may be able, in some sense, to speak to the more "usual" personality, even though he or she will not reply to you in the moment. Be warned that this technique may make you feel a little crazy, but you can, if you desire to, gently or even humorously say something such as "I know the person I usually talk to is in there somewhere, and I'd like to spend some time with him when he comes back." A seemingly bizarre remark of this nature is often received matter-of-factly by someone with a dissociative identity disorder, as if it made perfect sense. Bear in mind that he will not reply to your statement immediately, may never overtly reply to it at all, but there can be comfort, especially when you care about the person who has switched, in feeling that you have made a connection, even if brief and unconventional.

And how would someone know if he himself were a switcher?

The human need for consistency and safety being what it is, switching is easily misinterpreted, explained away, or simply disavowed, and its invisibility to us makes us vulnerable to a legion of interpersonal and social problems. But having said this, let me point out that there are signs, theoretically discernible as private experience, for those who are truly interested in beginning to assess themselves:

Like Nathan, a switcher experiences time distortions and time lapses, which he or she has probably spent years consciously trying to rationalize and excuse. Other people sometimes tell him of significant things he has done for which he realizes he has no memory, whether he publicly confesses his amnesia or not. From his companions, he receives descriptions (the way Lars the Liar did from his wife) of extreme changes they have observed in him. These observations may be accompanied by angry complaints, or tearful entreaties to explain, or to desist. Like Camisha, someone who switches may sense that she is causing emotional pain for people she cares about, though she genuinely does not comprehend why or how this is happening. Or like Sarah with her suicide cache, she may find completed or half-completed projects, purchased items, or handwriting among her personal effects that she cannot explain to herself, or even recognize.

To her bafflement, friends may claim that she is impossible to get close to, or that she is secretive, or unbearably silent at times. She may hear voices in her head, although she knows better than to admit this experience to anyone. These voices tend to comment upon her actions, and are sometimes so clamorous, and so at odds with each other, that she is temporarily immobilized.

If most or all of this feels familiar—or, I should add, if merely trying to think about the above makes the reader feel strangely sleepy or phased out—then a person may justifiably wonder about dissociative identity disorder as a factor in his or her own psychological makeup. Such a person, one who is brave enough to wonder about himself or herself in this way, is unusual and commendable indeed. And if you have come far enough to pose these questions, I commend you, and I urge you to find an excellent therapist, and allow her to help you become, in time, the integrated person you richly deserve to be.

In fact, if you have come this bold distance already, healing (with help) is not only possible. It is likely.

And now for the rest of us. Though more people suffer from DID than we understand, certainly we are not all multiple, or otherwise profoundly dissociative. We do not all try to save others from the

Coconut Grove nightclub fire, or provoke them to reenact the jungle combat we survived decades ago. We do not all turn into innocent little children again, like Brooke, or perform unaccountable (and unremembered) feats of strength, like Meng, or fail to recognize the clothes we are wearing or the handwriting we have produced, or terrorize our families, or fall into an altered state and set out to police the night.

However, we are, all of us, mildly to moderately dissociative, and if we look closely, we can see the signs of this in ourselves. Imagine a list, not formally a continuum, but something that does tend to increase in severity, or perhaps "detachment from self," as it progresses. At the top of the list are nontrauma items such as daydreaming and movie-watching, relatively uncomplicated states of mind we can all recognize. At the bottom is trauma's most elaborate handiwork: dissociative identity disorder, like Nathan's or Garrett's.

And in the middle of the list are the following:

Brief phasing out. This readily happens to us in situations that involve performance anxiety (speaking in public, appearing in an important ceremony such as a wedding, etc.), or after accidents (car crashes, for example) or even near-accidents. Brief phasing out—momentarily departing from present experience—may or may not include a short-lived sense of being out-of-body and watching from a distance, and sometimes results in small gaps in one's memory, or a temporary sense that time has collapsed. (Where did the day go? What did I do this afternoon anyway? Oh, there was that bicyclist I almost hit. . . .)

Habitual dissociative reactions. These are the repeated mental absences exhibited by Matthew, the "space cadet." A person who displays such reactions will often have nicknames or labels bestowed upon him by others—"absentminded," "in your own little world," "introvert," or even "passive-aggressive." If you frequently lose your place in a conversation, or in a day, and especially if you do this to the point that others notice and remark, you may be exhibiting habitual dissociative reactions. In addition, you may receive complaints from those closest to you that you are ignoring them, or that, in their opinion, you will not "face" or "deal with" certain issues, usually emotional ones.

Dissociation from feeling states. This was Grandma Cleo when she met her first grandchild, after an uncomfortably anxious time just before his birth. Typically, this dissociative reaction is marked by feeling nothing at all, though the individual may be intellectually aware, during or perhaps after the fact, that feelings are called for.

Or, this form of dissociation may involve a lifelong cordoning off and dispossession of the "dangerous" emotion of anger. Beyond mere rules for behavior during conflict—"I must not show my anger"—this reaction is genuinely experienced and sometimes expressed as "I never get angry," or "I really can't remember the last time I got angry." This, ironically, can make the people around one very angry indeed, for its apparent "dishonesty."

Intrusion of dissociated ego states. Kenneth was intruded upon by a dissociated ego state when he visited the airy heights of the World Trade Center's observation deck with his first-grade son. Normally optimistic and friendly, for a few hours after his trip Kenneth felt strangely vigilant and mean-spirited, for no apparent reason. The intrusion of a dissociated ego state is, in a certain way, the converse of the dissociation of a feeling state; instead of having one's own emotions yanked away to leave a vacancy, one's usual feeling patterns and attitudes are temporarily tainted and muddled by the entrance of an extra "personality," an anonymous part of one's mental makeup that is most often silent.

Dissociated ego states that intrude are typically angry, self-protective, and uneasily suspicious and accusatory of other people. When a person is influenced in this way, he may feel uncomfortable about his hostility during the episode, confused, or even mildly alarmed. The dissociative reaction is sometimes accompanied by unspoken thoughts such as, "Why am I so angry at the world all of a sudden? This doesn't make any sense. I think I'd better chill out."

However, deliberate chilling out is not really an option; such a state seems to arrive and depart on its own obscure terms.

Demifugue. Lila, who told me about becoming her "flyaway self" because a cashier was rude to her, and Seth, who described how he would mentally drift out to a lonely gray sea whenever he was triggered, were both reporting the occurrence of demifugue. Demifugue imposes a generalized detachment from self and others, a mental and emotional fogginess that seems to have a life of its own. The fog can be thin and annoying, or it can be an anesthetizing pea-souper. Some people know this state as intensely frustrating, and other people experience it as comforting and safe.

In addition to fogginess or gauziness, people describe demifugue in various ways. Some speak of being trapped on the wrong end of a telescope; the whole world seems unreachably far away and small. Or some feel overwhelmed by fatigue, defeated by it—"I can't even keep my eyes open"—no matter how much rest and sleep they take.

Or—and this is potentially the most damaging manifestation of demifugue—there can be a near-complete rift in body/mind communication, and thus in the individual's capacity to discern her own serious pain, illness, or injury. This is what happened to Julia when she did not feel pain from her ruptured appendix, and proceeded to lose consciousness altogether. Such a separation between body and mind is not the same thing as the characteristic we usually refer to as a "high tolerance for pain," which is just that, a tolerance, and a fortunate one when pain must be consciously endured. When significant pain is not perceived at all, or is dismissed as unimportant, this is not "tolerance," but is probably the result, instead, of a moderate-to-severe dissociative state.

Fugue. Beyond distance and grayness, fugue is a total blackout. Julia had been in a fugue when, for example, she woke up on what she thought was a Tuesday morning, and later discovered it was a Friday. During fugue, one's life often appears, from the outside, to go on more or less as usual. The self-aware "center"—the part that wishes, dreams, has emotions, and remembers—takes flight; but certain intellectually driven functions remain, converse almost as usual with others, carry out the normal tasks.

What occurs during fugue is not remembered by the person later (dissociative amnesia), and those who suffer fugue have the experience of "losing time," hours, days, weeks, and sometimes even longer.

These six dissociative reactions comprise the middle part of the list, sandwiched between daydreaming and switching, and there is something for everyone here. Protracted trauma-related fugue is not a frequent occurrence for most of us. But demifugue is fairly common. We tend to be *triggered* (involuntarily propelled) into the fog of a demifugue by events that somehow pose a threat to our *physical integrity*, to our sense of *being in control*, or to our relationships (ah yes, especially our *relationships*). And to a degree, after we become savvy to them, we can predict certain triggers in ourselves, and anticipate them in other people, so that patience and kind treatment (for others and for ourselves) become more likely.

Most of these triggering events are, in actuality, not very earth-shaking. In terms of threat to physical integrity, receiving scary medical or dental news can be a trigger, unsurprisingly—but so can a radical haircut. Our sense of being in control can be assaulted, and our consciousness muddled, by minor financial jolts (e.g., the loan refusal comes in the mail), or by even small changes in our work settings—"I got to work and they had moved my desk!"—or by sudden disruptions in our customary means of getting to where we want to go: the car breaks down, the airport is closed. A subway strike, for instance, can launch multitudes of people into brief hazy-eyed demifugue, all at the same time.

Changes, in general, tend to trigger us into dissociative behavior, especially if they are unexpected.

As for our relationships—we are all easily triggered by evaluations, perceived rejections, and especially discord. In fact, if you want to know what dissociation feels like, the next time you have a serious argument with someone who is meaningful to you—your employer or your parent or your spouse—pick up a newspaper or a book; sit and read for a while. And an hour or two later, try with all your might to recall what you read.

It was Mark Twain who said, "When we remember that we are all mad, the mysteries disappear and life stands explained." Perhaps recognizing this is the first step toward feeling compassion, for ourselves and for other people too, when we temporarily absent ourselves from our own minds. We are in this together. We all have a few faulty fuses. And so the question is not *Who?* but rather *How?*

How do we take responsibility? How do we fix it?

CHAPTER NINE

As It Should Be

All sanity is great madness, but the greatest madness of
all is to live life the way it is, rather than as it should be.

—Cervantes

A trauma survivor desiring lasting change must confront moments in which she feels an irresistible urge to run from the process of remembering, feels inexcusably stupid, in fact, for not heeding the shrill warnings of her own mind to abandon the attempt, to flee; and set upon by these intolerable feelings, she must nonetheless stand her ground. Repelled though she may feel, she must continue to stare directly into the face of the past, to see it as clearly as possible, to describe it in words, to attach names to the nameless emotional monsters that have promised to devour her should they ever be allowed to raise their heads above the amygdala bog.

Garrett, a real-life hero, has provided me with many piercing illustrations of this struggle. Sometimes, one of Garrett's dissociated ego states would be elected to express the excruciating nature of the dilemma. Near the end of his second year in therapy with me, for example, the alter personality "Abe" spoke in session for the first time, while Garrett himself was hypnotized.

"Abe" was the alter apparently in charge of handling all the grief, feelings of culpability, and paralyzing shame associated with the murder of Garrett's younger brother, Lef, which was committed by the boys' uncle when Garrett was ten years old. Inside, "Abe" harangued Garrett mercilessly, insisting that amends must be made in the form of Garrett's own death. Garrett must commit suicide; no other outcome was conscionable. And when "Abe" was in charge, he would sometimes make alarming headway toward this outcome, acquiring gun and bullets, and be thwarted in the act only by a dangerously ambivalent recapture of control by Garrett.

I believed that Garrett would benefit by "letting 'Abe' out" in therapy. But Garrett let me know that "Abe" was issuing dire warnings against the possibility. "Abe" advised us both that should he be allowed "out" in my office, something disastrous would take place, something dreadful and ugly that neither Garrett nor I would be able to bear. "Abe" shouted inside Garrett's mind, in exhortations that became frequent and despairing, that unmeetable danger was looming, and that Garrett was on the verge of a deadly mistake.

When Garrett finally did switch to "Abe" during an hypnosis session, he sobbingly "confessed" to having murdered his little brother, Lef. In a long, soul-racking tirade that was grueling even to listen to, "Abe" tried to describe fragments of sensory memory that he had tragically come to label as "how it feels to kick a six-year-old child to death":

"I can feel my toes squashing into his side. *Squash! Squash! Squash!* Now he's making little noises. Oh Lef, be quiet! Stop it! Stop it!"

His poet's face was distorted in a wild grimace. He held his hands over his ears, and rocked his bone-thin body back and forth. Then, suddenly, he sat still and stared wide-eyed into space, as if he had just seen the gates into (and out of) a fiery hell.

"No. It's Uncle Dean. Uncle Dean is kicking him. It's not me. I don't think it's me. Oh God! Stop it! Stop it! Please, oh please, *please!* I'll be good. I'll be good. I promise. I promise."

During this session, and three additional ones, "Abe" continued this writhing, pleading, who-is-kicking-Lef debate with himself, in which the stakes were literally life-and-death for Garrett. In the end, "Abe" rendered an astonished final judgment of not guilty upon the psychologically mangled ten-year-old boy whom Garrett had been; but this irresolute epiphany came only after he had, with me as witness, repeatedly suffered the agonies of the damned.

Following "Abe's" four appearances in my office, he began to go away. Two months later, Garrett said he could no longer "sense 'Abe'," although he was not sure where "Abe" had gone. At about this time, Garrett started to acquire conscious memories of having witnessed his brother's murder, an event for which Garrett himself had previously been completely amnesic. Prior to these new memories, he had known about the murder only because he had been told, and because of the police and court proceedings that had surrounded the crime.

The memories inaugurated another painful process for Garrett: describing that same traumatic afternoon in coherent words, to himself and to me. Two narrative-constructing sessions were consumed in wrenching flashbacks and uncontrollable sobbing. During the first of these hours, he was forced to rush out of the session, because he had to vomit in the bathroom. But at the end of all this, Garrett no longer had a monstrous hidden memory. He had, instead, a monstrous explicit (or "declarative") memory, and this has made all the difference, as his therapy, and his life, have continued to unfold.

Of course, his verbal memory of the day Lef died is constructed, imperfect, after the fact. But so is all verbal memory whatsoever.

As I write this book, Garrett is still in therapy with me, and will probably be in treatment for some time to come. But he is much better, by his standards and also by mine. To his tremendous relief, he no longer switches in public, and is far less dissociative in general, with the notable exception that little "James" still "comes out" occasionally when Garrett is alone. My best prognosis is that eventually Garrett will not switch at all. To my own satisfaction, he has joined Alcoholics Anonymous, and no longer uses vodka, or any other anesthetizing substance. Even better, from my point of view, he has ruled out death by suicide as an option. He has decided to live.

He is now officially a member of Habitat for Humanity, because of what he describes as his "responsibility to help others in the world," and does house-painting and other work for that organization, stateside. He has become rather fluent in Spanish, and his dream is still to be "together enough" to travel to Central America someday. I believe this dream is within his reach.

Garrett's mother is still living, although his relationship with her is minimal. She resides on eastern Long Island, alone, in a small duplex near the Sound. He sends her money, and about twice a year, he drives down to pay what he refers to as his "conscience visits."

"Maybe she's glad to see me, maybe she's not. I can't really tell. She gives me tea. We sit in her little shoe box living room—I always feel like I won't fit. It's very . . . it's very neat, I guess you'd call it. There's no mess. And she uses a lot of those stick-up air freshener things. Smells like a rest room in a nice restaurant, is what it reminds me of, if you know what I mean.

"I never spend the night. It's just too depressing. All she has left in her life, seems like, is the damn TV, her doctor programs and her lawyer programs. You'd think she knew these people. She gives me tea, and we don't say anything at first—I can, like, hear my watch ticking—and then she'll ask me if I saw such-and-such a program on TV last night, and if I didn't—which I never have—she'll tell me all about it. As if I'd be interested in that, as if anyone's interested in that. Weirds me out.

"I try to get her to tell me what needs fixing around the place— it would make me feel better to do *something*—but she always tells me there's nothing. Which isn't true. Oh, and get this—about four or five years ago, she and the lady in the other half of the house had the place aluminum sided, so I can't even paint it for her."

Knowing what the answer probably was, I asked whether she ever spoke of Lef, her little son who was murdered. Garrett shook his head emphatically.

"No, no, she won't talk about him, not how he died or anything. What I mean is—she won't talk about him at all. If I even just bring up his name, she changes the subject. Starts telling me about *Law and Order* all over again, or whatever.

"When I get to the point where I really just can't stand it, I leave. She doesn't try to stop me. Six hours to drive down there, and another six hours back. Oh well."

Garrett is well on his way to triumphing over his dissociative disorder. But profound trauma makes more than one kind of cut into a person's life. Psychologically an orphan, undereducated, still deeply unsure of himself as a person, and understandably wary of other people, Garrett has a few "friends" with whom he socializes, but no one, as yet, who is genuinely close to him, no one who shares his most private thoughts, or his heart. I see him as a lonely, valiant human being still striving to be whole.

Garrett's is an extreme case, and his suffering was extraordinary. How about everyone else? How do the rest of us resolve our stories, bring more light and warmth and honest courage to our lives?

I suspect that the healing process in the real world closely parallels the therapeutic process in the session room, and that having another person, such as a therapist, along on the journey makes it inestimably easier. As for the journey itself, here are some pointers:

First of all, be as safe as possible in the present, literally. To my patients, I recommend a personal sanctuary, which is most often one's own home. Make your home a peaceful and secure place to go to, in every detail, beginning with a neighborhood that feels safe, and continuing to an especially appealing and comfortable bed. If locks on the door make you feel better, install lots of them.

Buy comforts. Keep a pet. Fall in love with silence.

Regardless of what your patterns may always have been, learn to separate yourself now—and again, literally—from difficult, crisis-addicted, rageful, and, most particularly, violent people. Keep as much social and physical distance between these people and your-self as you would between them and an innocent child in your care.

Have routines. Make them sacred. Sleep every night.

A nurtured, nontumultuous life tends to promote in a human creature the relatively serene hormonal and neurological environ-ment in which traumatic memory may be reclaimed. And this is the task at hand. Recovery involves the reprocessing of fragmented primitive memories into integrated conscious memories, and the reduction of outdated dissociative reactions. It requires hard, pre-carious, frightening *memory work*—a mosaic of activities, some-times including hypnosis, the consistent practice of meditation, the recording of dreams, and "detective" attempts such as looking up old records, visiting old places, talking with relatives, and ask-ing unwelcome questions that often lead to no very clear answers.

As you go along, keep a daily journal of your reactions, your thoughts, and your feelings.

Even with all this exertion, none of us will ever recall more than a fraction of all that has happened to us in the surge of a whole life-time, and even what we think we know for sure will be subject to our chattering self-doubts. Fortunately, providentially, remember-ing only a fraction of all that has happened will usually turn out to be just enough.

Of course, remembering some good things is important, as well. Human life is always mixed, and so are genuine memories of it.

In my practice, I often use hypnosis as an avenue to the consol-idation of memory, as I did with Garrett and with Julia. Progress made by an individual under hypnosis does not conform to the traditional notion of purging or "catharsis"; there is no instant elimination of harmful unconscious material simply because it is expressed consciously. The person does not suddenly say "Saints preserve us! So this is what happened!" and then have an intense emotional reaction (an "abreaction") that leads to an immediate breathtaking advance. More nearly, trance facilitates a progressive re-forming of memory on a deeper level than is ordinarily possible, a gradual two-steps-forward-one-step-back reworking that must occur in combination with other sources of information and support. As one component of treatment, hypnosis by a sensitive practitioner is productive and intriguing. However, it is by no means a sufficient or even a necessary approach to recovery.

Another excellent approach, again neither necessary nor sufficient—but definitely helpful—is the faithful practice of some form of meditation, an ancient and respected path. Two types that may be especially fruitful in memory work (and perhaps in the healing of *shin pan*) are Tibetan emptiness meditations, and a form of meditation that is most often referred to as "mindfulness."

When practiced devotedly, Tibetan meditations calm the mind; they promote stability of attention, and extremely deep states of mental peace. These meditations involve "one-pointed" concentration—what Westerners might call "emptying the mind"—and are what Buddhists call *shamantha* or *samadhi* practices. Mindfulness meditation, on the other hand, is sometimes called insight meditation, or *vipasana* meditation. *Vipasana* means, roughly, "to see things as they really are," and though mindfulness meditation usually begins with a "mind-emptying" technique to foster stability and calm, it then introduces the concept of observation, and a certain amount of inquiry into the unknown and the unclear. The essence of mindfulness meditation (which is perhaps most often associated with the Vietnamese Buddhist monk, teacher, and peacemaker, Thich Nhat Hanh) is a kind of silent witnessing, a dispassionate observing that helps the meditator to "see" what is on her mind, without altering it, censoring it, or being afraid of it.

I would like to emphasize that regardless of your practice—therapy, hypnosis, or meditation—memory consolidation does not happen all at once. Be exceedingly patient with yourself, like a kindly grandparent, as the Taoists say. Memory comes in fits and starts, and like Matthew when he suddenly reconsidered his mother's

insult, "You maggot!" we "remember" things by viewing them differently, by relabeling them, by sharing them with other people, at
least as often as we "remember" by calling forth entirely new facts.

The overall goal is to form a few regular memories, to use Julia's
term. Noteworthy is the fact that early in her work toward this
objective, Julia voiced a concern about its purpose. She could not
imagine that there was anything to be gained by "blaming other
people" for her problems. And in general, she found the entire notion of blaming to be offensive. She was not interested in assigning
blame to others, and did not want to spend any time on such a pur-
suit, even though she had begun to remember that her own parents
had tortured and humiliated her throughout her childhood, and
though the dominant culture around her—around us all—would
tolerate, even applaud self-involvement, finger-pointing, and re-
taliation.

"What good will it do to dwell on all this? I have to live my own
life now."

I told her, as I have told many others, that blaming is surely not
the point. The purpose of consolidating memories, and of making
them verbal, is not to figure out who was at fault. "Fault" is a peculiar concept anyway, and has no place in the healing process, except perhaps to affirm that the victim herself was *not* at fault. And
a preoccupation with blaming and avenging will blind a person to
her own self-discovery. Rather, the advantage of having regular
memories is in knowing, explicitly and as objectively as possible,
what has happened in one's life.

Consolidated memories, even horrible ones, are far better than
scraps of sensory memory that get stirred up at odd moments to
cause dissociative episodes. And explicit memory of life events is
better, too, because it is active and useful. Sensory images by themselves are static; introspection and discussion do not alter them one
whit, nor can they be employed as cognitive tools. As an illustration, if a person survives a plane crash, and afterward all that
remains in his mind of the traumatic experience is fragmented sen-

sory memory—disorganized and frightening images and sounds, and waves of unbearable emotion that assail him at unpredictable moments, or in nightmares—then he will be unable to ask important questions about the event.

Examples of important questions, both irrational and rational (both of which occur to trauma survivors) are, "Did the plane go down because I am a bad person?" and, "Will all planes crash?" and, "What effective precautions can I take if I ever get on a plane again?" Such questions can be asked, and discussed with other people, only if memory can be made explicit. And the answers are important not because one wants above all to know whether or not to blame the pilot. The answers are important, crucial, because one wishes no longer to have terrors at night, and debilitating dissociative experiences during the day.

The last question about the plane crash, the one about future precautions, is especially significant, because it exposes a traitorous incongruity: the fact that after trauma has passed, dissociative reactions do not protect us. On the contrary, they place us at much greater risk. Fragmented memory and knee-jerk dissociative behaviors leave us unable to think things through, perilously ill-equipped to problem-solve, or to respond effectively to present and future dangers, or even to understand when we are safe. This feature of dissociative capacity is its largest and most regrettable irony. The irony affects individual people such as Garrett and Julia and you and me, as well as people in collectives, such as families, subcultures, nations. Unable to think our way through to a constructive plan, we persist in the familiar, the same old tactics, though they have previously shown themselves to be ineffective, sometimes even destructive and painful.

The true remedies are making a safe place, finding out, remembering, not hiding from the memories, and not blaming. Also, at first, simply learning to recognize dissociative behavior in oneself and in others, at least some of the time, may be counted as a part of the cure. By definition, increased self-observation exercises the observing ego, the part of the self that will be able to view dissociation as a currently unnecessary limit upon one's freedom.

These are difficult prescriptions, and as I say, the presence of another person, a therapist or a mentor, is helpful, may even be required. But the alternative is for us to continue in something reminiscent of a tedious science fiction plot in which the otherwise admirable characters are trapped in an hermetic time loop, and repeat over and over again the same galaxy-shattering mistakes, never ascertaining that they have done it all a fathomless number of times before. In this sort of plot, the only way out is somehow to perceive and sever the time loop, of which the only detectable symptom is a wispy sense of *déjà vu*.

The survival-programmed dissociative function of our brains is not the only arena in which human beings must ultimately take a stand against their own biologically prepared nature. Hardship and survival of the fittest through the ages have endowed us with hormonally aggressive temperaments, and us-them wiring, the law-of-the-jungle logic of which is no more astute than "He is different. Kill him." This wiring is the basis of violence seemingly without limit, and nearly all hatred, vengeance-taking, prejudice, bigotry, and other archaic predispositions that now make us miserable upon our own planet, and that have directed our history as a perpetually traumatized group.

We are a young species, evolutionarily speaking, and the phenomenon of conscious awareness, supposedly our claim to fame, is extremely new to us. We are bare beginners at it. In essence, human beings are transcendent spirits housed inside freshly evolved brains that are trying to deal with the same old earthly realities as loggerhead turtles, that our bodies and the bodies of our lifelong companions are soon broken and empty, and even our beautiful children may not survive. Looked at in this way, it is miraculous that we have endured.

Like any other species that has ever been around, we have passed a survival test, at least for the moment. The uniquely human question is not, "Can we adapt to trauma and survive?" but is instead, "Can we now overcome our memories of trauma, and learn truly to live?" Such a development would mark a new and higher plane of human functioning altogether. And if we are to continue at all, the transition may have to come relatively soon, perhaps even within this new millennium.

In my work, I have seen some extraordinary individuals make this change, against unreasonable odds, and in spite of having been hurt in ways that most of us would have trouble imagining. Julia is one of these people. As I write, Julia is no longer in weekly therapy. Two years ago, she graduated, in a manner of speaking, and I now see her only occasionally, once every few months, for "tune-ups," as she calls them. In the last two years, she has married, bought a house, taken up skiing, and has produced several new documentary films, one of these on the recognition and prevention of child abuse.

She still has not moved back to Los Angeles for her career. "Someday maybe," she says, and then she usually changes the subject.

She does not lose time anymore. She no longer wishes to die. To the contrary, she is expecting her first child.

I saw her most recently on a warm afternoon last October, when she came to my office for one of her scheduled "tune-ups."

"Guess what!" she greeted me, still standing, her back to my little Haitian figurine.

"What?" I asked.

"I'm six weeks pregnant! I found out for sure yesterday."

"Oh my God!"

She hugged me, and we both almost cried.

Wearing sandals and a blue linen sheath, she stood in the middle of the room, and announced that she had driven to Boston directly from a morning at the beach. Her hair was longer than I had ever seen it, and was not quite contained in a narrow silver headband.

"I went to the beach where I tried to kill myself that time. . . ."

"Why?" I interrupted, alarmed.

"No, no. Not to worry. This time I went just because it's so peaceful there. I figured I might have missed some of the scenery when I was busy trying to off myself."

She smiled at me, obviously amused at her own sly humor. I raised my eyebrows.

"That could be," I said.

"No, really, it's wonderful there, unbelievable. I mean, I've been to beaches so many times in my life, but today it was like I was there for the very first time. It was like I'd just discovered it. I walked and I walked and I walked. And then I turned around and looked back, and of course I saw my own footprints. They went back just as far as I could see, back and back. It was so moving, I don't know exactly how to explain it. Nothing else, just this gorgeous, empty beach. It smells so *good!* I wanted to breathe it all in, all of it! I felt like I never wanted to leave. Have you ever felt like that?"

Not waiting for me to answer, she continued excitedly, "I know it's October, but I took off my shoes and started wading in the water. You know, if you stand at the edge and let the little waves go in and out over your feet, the sand kind of trickles away, and you feel like you're moving. You're really standing in one place, but the ocean makes you feel like you're moving, like you're gliding. Makes you feel like raising your arms and just gliding all the way to Portugal!"

She gazed at her feet, and lifted her arms like wings, as if in demonstration.

Trauma makes more than one kind of cut. I thought of Julia's unbearable past, and I knew that, even though she had overcome her dissociative disorder, her happiness would often be tempered by loneliness and grief—as it is for us all. But on this afternoon, to my delight, the room contained only a celebration, and one unattended, for now, by either fear or pain. Parenthood, sane and nonabusive parenthood, requires being present in the moment (at least most of the time . . .) with a new soul whom one introduces to the world. And during this hour, after her years of achingly hard work, Julia and I could celebrate her being able to do this.

The buck, uncounted generations of childhood trauma in Julia's family, had stopped with Julia.

She put down her wings, looked at me again, and said, "Have I mentioned that I'm pregnant?"

I laughed.

Finally, we settled into the familiar leather chairs, she took a deep breath, and we talked. Her voice was full of merriment, almost musical, no longer anything at all like the voice of a detached film narrator for her own life. She told me about taking the pregnancy test, and about her husband's reaction the previous evening, which had been as joyful as her own. We talked about her age, because the mother-to-be was nearly forty by now.

And of course, we talked about the future.

"Do you think the baby will have your auburn hair?"

She grinned, and answered, "I don't know. Paul's very dark. But one thing I do know is that she'll have her mother. I'll be right there with her, in the present, all the time. That's really the best gift I can give her, I think."

There was a pause while Julia considered.

Then she went on. "Oh, and when she can walk, I'm going to take her to the beach and show her that thing about the waves. It's so amazing."

I looked at her in admiration.

"Amazing," I agreed.

NOTES

CHAPTER TWO

page 18: *A growing body of research:* Most notably by Joseph LeDoux of New York University, and by Bessel van der Kolk, Roger Pitman, and Scott Rauch of Harvard Medical School. See J. LeDoux, "Emotion as Memory: Anatomical Systems Underlying Indelible Neural Traces," in S.-A. Christianson (ed.), *Handbook of Emotion and Memory*, Hillsdale, N.J.: Erlbaum, 1992; B. van der Kolk, "The Body Keeps the Score: Memory and the Evolving Psychobiology of PTSD," *Harvard Review of Psychiatry, 1* (1994), 253–265; R. Pitman, "The Black Hole of Trauma," *Biological Psychiatry, 26* (1990), 221–223; and S. Rauch, B. van der Kolk, R. Fisler, N. Alpert, S. Orr, C. Savage, A. Fischman, M. Jenike, and R. Pitman, "A Symptom Provocation Study of Posttraumatic Stress Disorder Using Positron Emission Tomography and Script-driven Imagery," *Archives of General Psychiatry, 53* (1996), 380–387.

CHAPTER THREE

page 51:   *Child abuse, as in Julia's case:* In 1989, the federal government established the National Child Abuse and Neglect Data System (NCANDS), a voluntary data collection and analysis system. Each year, NCANDS, under the sponsorship of the Children's Bureau in the Administration of Children, Youth and Families of the U.S. Department of Health and Human Services, makes data available for use by the research community. The summary data component of this annual report provides aggregate counts from all fifty states on items such as the number of children who were the subject of a maltreatment report, the number of child victims, and the age and race of the child victims. These data are available through the National Clearinghouse on Child Abuse and Neglect Information, Washington, D.C. For information on sexual abuse specifically, see David Finkelhor's excellent work, *A Sourcebook on Child Sexual Abuse*, Newbury Park, Calif.: Sage, 1986.

page 51:   *For children to witness violence:* See *Domestic Violence for Health Care Providers*, 3rd edition, Denver: Colorado Domestic Violence Coalition, 1991; and J. Osofsky, "The Effects of Exposure to Violence on Young Children," *American Psychologist*, 50 (1995), 782–788.

page 52:   *One of the most widely accepted and helpful definitions:* A. McFarlane and G. de Girolamo, "The Nature of Traumatic Stressors and the Epidemiology of Posttraumatic Reactions," in B. van der Kolk, A. McFarlane, and L. Weisaeth (eds.), *Traumatic Stress: The Effects of Overwhelming Experience on Mind, Body, and Society*, New York: Guilford Press, 1996.

CHAPTER FOUR

page 70:   *During World War II:* Regarding the use of hypnosis in the treatment of trauma survivors from World War II to the present, see J. Watkins, "The Psychodynamic Treatment of Combat Neuroses (PTSD) with Hypnosis during World War II," *International Journal of Clinical and Experimental Hypnosis, 48* (2000), 324–335; R. Kluft, "The Use of Hypnosis with Dissociative Disorders," *Psychiatric Medicine, 10* (1992), 31–46; D. Spiegel, "The Use of Hypnosis in the Treatment of PTSD," *Psychiatric Medicine, 10* (1992), 21–30; and D. Spiegel, "Hypnosis in the Treatment of Victims of Sexual Abuse," *Psychiatric Clinics of North America, 12* (1989), 295–305. For detailed descriptions of some hypnotic techniques in the treatment of dissociative disorders, see M. Phillips and C. Frederick, *Healing the Divided Self: Clinical and Ericksonian Hypnotherapy for Post-Traumatic and Dissociative Conditions,* London: W.W. Norton and Company, 1995.

page 75: *So, what are the available facts?:* For a discussion of the most commonly reported triggers for the recall of traumatic events, see D. Elliott, "Traumatic Events: Prevalence and Delayed Recall in the General Population," *Journal of Consulting and Clinical Psychology, 65* (1997), 811–820.

page 76: *Regarding brain activity itself:* See J. Bremner, J. Krystal, D. Charney, and S. Southwick, "Neural Mechanisms in Dissociative Amnesia for Childhood Abuse: Relevance to the Current Controversy Surrounding the 'False Memory Syndrome'," *American Journal of Psychiatry, 153* (1996), 71–82.

page 76: *In addition to knowledge gained from neuroscience:* L. Williams, "Recall of Childhood Trauma: A Prospective Study of Women's Memories of Child Sexual Abuse," *Journal of Consulting and Clinical Psychology, 62* (1994), 1167–1176; and L. Williams, "Recovered Memories of Abuse in Women with Documented Child Sexual Victimization Histories," *Journal of Traumatic Stress, 8* (1995), 649–673.

page 102: *To illustrate the limitations of consciousness:* T. Nørretranders, *The User Illusion: Cutting Consciousness Down to Size,* New York: Viking, 1998.

CHAPTER FIVE

page 117:　*As with our depersonalized bride: Depersonalization* is a sense of detachment from the self, as opposed to *derealization* (Seth out on his ocean, for example), which is a sense that one's surroundings are unreal. Depersonalization and derealization are two of the five components of dissociation that are considered to be systematically measurable. The other three are amnesia, identity confusion, and identity alteration. For a discussion of these components and of how they are measured, see M. Steinberg, "Systematizing Dissociation: Symptomatology and Diagnostic Assessment," in D. Spiegel (ed.), *Dissociation: Culture, Mind, and Body*, Washington, D.C.: American Psychiatric Press, 1994.

CHAPTER SIX

page 140:　*Though I had hedged a little:* This 1646 description by Paracelsus is cited by E. Bliss, in "Multiple Personalities: A Report of 14 Cases with Implications for Schizophrenia and Hysteria," *Archives of General Psychiatry, 37* (1980), 1388–1397.

page 141:　*Emotional embroilments notwithstanding:* Three such standardized assessment measures are the Dissociative Disorders Interview Schedule, the Dissociative Experiences Scale, and the Structured Clinical Interview for DSM-IV Dissociative Disorders. Cross-cultural studies include C. Ross, S. Miller, P. Reagor, L. Bjornson, G. Fraser, and G. Anderson, "Structured Interview Data on 102 Cases of Multiple Personality Disorder from Four Centers," *American Journal of Psychiatry, 147* (1990), 596–601; S. Boon and N. Draijer, "Multiple Personality Disorder in The Netherlands: A Clinical Investigation of 71 Patients," *American Journal of Psychiatry, 150* (1993), 489–494: and V. Sar, L. Yargic, and H. Tutkun, "Structured Interview Data on 35 Cases of Dissociative Identity Disorder in Turkey," *American Journal of Psychiatry, 153* (1996), 1329–1333.

page 141:   *A report from the National Institute of Mental Health:* F. Putnam, "Recent Research on Multiple Personality Disorder," *Psychiatric Clinics of North America, 14* (1991), 489–502.

page 148:   *And Garrett desperately needed:* A fascinating discussion of research on death from helplessness, including C.P. Richter's findings, is to be found in Martin Seligman's groundbreaking work, *Helplessness: On Depression, Development, and Death,* San Francisco: W.H. Freeman and Company, 1975.

page 153:   *Cultural influences shape dissociative identity disorder:* See V. Varma, M. Bouri, and N. Wig, "Multiple Personality in India: Comparison with Hysterical Possession State," *American Journal of Psychotherapy, 35* (1981), 113–120; Adityanjee, G. Raju, and S. Khandelwal, "Current Status of Multiple Personality Disorder in India," *American Journal of Psychiatry, 146* (1989), 1607–1610; R. Castillo, "Spirit Possession in South Asia, Dissociation or Hysteria? Part 1: Theoretical Background," *Culture, Medicine and Psychiatry, 18* (1994), 1–21; R. Castillo, "Spirit Possession in South Asia, Dissociation or Hysteria? Part 2: Case Histories," *Culture, Medicine and Psychiatry, 18* (1994), 141–162; and A. Gaw, Q. Ding, R. Levine, and H. Gaw, "The Clinical Characteristics of Possession Disorder among 20 Chinese Patients in the Hebei Province of China," *Psychiatric Services, 49* (1998), 360–365.

CHAPTER SEVEN

page 162:   *In traditional personality studies:* Regarding what Walter Mischel refers to as "constructed consistencies" in observed behavior, three classic texts in psychology may be of interest: L. Festinger, *A Theory of Cognitive Dissonance,* Stanford, Calif.: Stanford University Press, 1957; P. Warr and C. Knapper, *The Perception of People and Events,* London: Wiley, 1968; and his own work, W. Mischel, *Personality and Assessment,* New York: Wiley, 1968.

page 162:   *If Kenneth's protective ego state begins to erupt much more often:*
The repeated but incomplete intrusion of Kenneth's dissoci-
ated ego state is a type of reaction that the *Diagnostic and Statistical Manual of Mental Disorders IV* classifies with a
somewhat ambiguous term, "dissociative disorder not otherwise specified" (DDNOS), rather than the more definitive
"dissociative identity disorder" (DID).

CHAPTER EIGHT

page 201:   *The dissociative nature of our consciousness:* The case study of
Melody D. can be found in B. van der Kolk and W. Kadish,
"Amnesia, Dissociation, and the Return of the Repressed," in
B. van der Kolk (ed.), *Psychological Trauma*, Washington,
D.C.: American Psychiatric Press, 1987. The case study of
the Vietnam veteran can be found in B. van der Kolk, "The
Compulsion To Repeat Trauma: Revictimization, Attach-
ment and Masochism," *Psychiatric Clinics of North America, 12*
(1989), 389–411.

page 210:   *Countless writers, philosophers, and yes, even scientists:* The story
of Jimmie G. can be found as "The Lost Mariner," in O.
Sacks, *The Man Who Mistook His Wife for a Hat and Other
Clinical Tales*, New York: Summit Books, 1985.

page 218:   *However, we are, all of us, mildly to moderately dissociative:* The
idea that the dissociative reactions might form a continuum
of some kind has occurred independently to a number of cli-
nicians and researchers, and the available research would
seem to support a continuum model. See S. Boon and N.
Draijer, *Multiple Personality Disorder in The Netherlands*, Am-
sterdam: Swets and Zeitlinger, 1993; P. Coons, "Dissociative
Disorder Not Otherwise Specified: A Clinical Investigation
of 50 Cases with Suggestions for Typology and Treatment,"
Dissociation, 5 (1992), 187–195; and C. Ross, G. Anderson, G.
Fraser, P. Reagor, L. Bjornson, and S. Miller, "Differentiat-

ing Multiple Personality Disorder and Dissociative Disorder Not Otherwise Specified," *Dissociation*, 5 (1992), 88–91.

CHAPTER NINE

page 229:   *Another excellent approach:* See for example, Thich Nhat Hanh and Mobi Ho (trans.), *The Miracle of Mindfulness: A Manual on Meditation*, Boston: Beacon Press, 1996.

INDEX

abandonment, 55–58
abortion, 94–97
abreaction, 228–29
absentmindedness, 19–20, 105–13,
   147, 160–61, 194–95, 218–19
abuse, child, *see* child abuse
accidents, 8, 19, 28, 51, 218, 230–31
acting, 22, 93, 98, 196–98
addiction, 109, 131
affect toleration, 71
aggressor, identification with, 90–91,
   203–4, 212–14
Alcoholics Anonymous, 226
alcoholism, 149, 160, 210–11, 226
alexithymia, 202–3
allergens, 147
American Psychiatric Association, 139
American Psychological Association,
   51
amnesia, 76, 188, 195, 201–2, 207–8,
   210–11, 215–17, 220–21, 225,
   240n
Amy (case study), 55, 58–60, 62
amygdala, 17, 76, 223
analgesia, 50, 85

anger, 19, 106, 111, 125–26, 154–55,
   170–72, 195, 202, 207, 219–20
animal magnetism, 68–69
Año Nuevo State Reserve, 47–49
anorexia nervosa, 10–11
anxiety, 54, 91, 114–17, 139–40, 164,
   179, 202, 204, 218
asthma, 147

baby talk, 186–87
Bambi, 54, 55
behavior:
   acceptable, 159–64, 215–16
   aggressive, 147
   consistent, 159–64, 208–10, 215–16,
      241n
   dissociative, *see* dissociation
   models for, 184–86
   unpredictable, 102–3, 168–70,
      174–77, 195
Bernhardt, Sarah, 196
Beverly (case study), 17–20, 117
"black belt," 153
blood glucose, 147
Boston Globe, 187

Braid, James, 69
brain, physiology of, 17–18, 19, 20,
    76, 147–48, 210–11, 223
breast cancer, 186
Breuer, Joseph, 70
Broca's area, 17–18
Brooke (case study), 186–87, 204,
    218
Buddhism, 229

Camisha (case study), 177–79, 196–97,
    198, 217
Carroll, Lewis, 15
catharsis, 228–29
Cervantes, Miguel de, 223
change, 221–22
Charcot, Jean-Martin, 69–70
Charlie (case study), 179–83,
    193–94
child abuse:
    admissions of, 204–8
    chronic, 76, 149, 163
    perpetuation of, 90–91, 209–10,
        234–35
    physical, 13, 25, 88–91, 143–44,
        147, 149, 191–93, 230
    prevalence of, 51–52, 55, 165,
        238n
    prevention of, 51, 233, 234–35
    psychological, 89–90, 144
    sexual, 10, 13–14, 73–76, 89–90,
        143–44, 147, 149, 163, 177,
        189–90, 204–8
children:
    cognitive capabilities of, 54–55
    curiosity of, 47–49
    fears of, 3–4, 49, 54–62, 85, 125–27,
        148–49, 184–85, 190, 203
    reality as perceived by, 30–31
"chilling out," 219–20
China, 153–54, 155
choc nerveux, 70
Cleo (case study), 128–31, 159–60,
    164, 219

Coconut Grove fire (1942), 201–2,
    217–18
cognitive restructuring, 71
combat stress, 28, 31–32, 70, 76
compartmentalization, 100–101,
    166–68, 207–9
compassion, 222
computers, 102
concentration, 38
congestive heart failure, 10–11
Conrad, Joseph, 3
consciousness, 74, 100, 101–2, 125–26
"constructed consistencies," 241n
control, 12, 106, 214–15, 221
cortex, 18
Così fan tutte (Mozart), 69
creativity, 114, 175–77
"crisis room," 68
cross-cultural studies, 141
Crystal (case study), 137–39
"cutting," 9–10, 137

daydreams, 27, 218
death, 53, 57, 58, 59, 109, 129, 148–49
defenses, mental, 5
de Girolamo, Giovanni, 52–53, 54
demifugue, 35–36, 123–24, 128, 160,
    217, 220, 221
depersonalization, 116–17, 240n
depression, 4, 13, 20, 21, 22, 62,
    64–66, 91, 94–97, 109, 126, 136,
    145, 146, 148, 164, 202
derealization, 36, 240n
Diagnostic and Statistical Manual of
    Mental Disorders IV (DSM IV),
    139, 146–47, 242n
Dickens, Charles, 176
disappearances, 168–70, 175, 178
dissociation:
    capacity for, 26–28, 30–31, 76, 131,
        218–19
    experience of, 25–26, 37–41,
        114–15, 131, 190–91, 193–94
    fugue and, 32–36, 220–21

hypnosis and, 69–70, 71, 91–103
process of, 5–9, 18–20, 58, 69–70, 71
severity of, 104–31, 217–21, 242n
as survival mechanism, 47–66, 100–101, 108
triggers for, 17–20, 35–36, 106–7, 112, 127, 131, 162, 201–2, 221
violence and, 183–86
see also ego states; fugue
dissociative disorder not otherwise specified (DDNOS), 242n
dissociative identity disorder (DID):
   cultural factors in, 153–56, 212–14, 230
   degrees of, 217–21, 242n
   diagnosis of, 127, 137, 139–42, 146–47, 148, 165, 240n, 242n
   invisibility of, 145–46, 148, 149, 154–55, 173, 177–79, 193–99
   popular misconceptions about, 140–41, 196, 197
   symptoms of, 146–50, 202–3, 208–9
   see also specific case studies
distraction, 26–28, 35, 194–95, 218
divorce, 109, 110–11
Dr. Jekyll/Mr. Hyde, 196
domestic violence, 51, 60–62, 187–88
Dorsett, Sybil Isabel, 197
dreams, 64–66, 73, 109, 121–22, 147
drugs, 131, 149
Duvalier, Baby Doc, 122
Dylan (case study), 55–58, 62

eating disorders, 10–11, 109
ego:
   alter, 203
   observing, 127–28, 130–31, 150, 163, 165, 194, 218, 220–21, 231–32
ego states:
   consistency of, 147–48, 209–10
   development of, 91–103, 126–27, 141, 147–48, 149, 162–64

dramatization of, 22, 93, 98, 196–98
intrusion of, 124–27, 219–20
naming of, 164–65, 195–96
switching of, 159–98, 202, 208, 209–10, 214–17, 223–27
see also specific case studies
Einstein, Albert, 114
emotions:
   cathartic, 228–29
   displays of, 106–7, 109
   lack of, 128–31, 166–68, 177, 178–79, 202–3, 219
   painful, 176–77, 216–17
   understanding of, 197, 202–3
   see also specific emotions
empathic perception, 197
"emptying the mind," 229
escape, 27
Esdaile, James, 69
estrangement, 125–26
"everyday misery," 5
exorcism, 154
eye contact, 95

families, 177–79, 193
fatigue, 123–24, 126, 128, 160, 217
fear, 3–4, 49, 54–62, 85, 125–27, 148–49, 184–85, 190, 203
feminism, 75, 186, 204
"fixity of gaze," 69
flashbacks, 17–20, 31–32, 117–23, 147, 225
"flyaway self," 35–36, 41, 220
Ford, Harrison, 26
forgetfulness, 19–20, 105–13, 147, 160–61, 194–95, 218–19
foster homes, 144
Frankl, Viktor, 135
Franklin, Benjamin, 68–69
free association, 70
French Academy of Sciences, 68–69
French-Indochinese War, 190–91
Freud, Sigmund, 5, 70, 74
Fugitive, The, 26–27, 28, 113–14

fugue, 32–36, 220–21
    demi-, 35–36, 123–24, 128, 160,
        217, 220, 221

Garrett (case study), 139–58
    Abe ego state of, 144–45, 150, 157,
        158, 223–25
    background of, 142–44
    "Big James" ego state of, 150, 157
    brother's death and, 144–45, 150,
        223–25, 227
    childhood trauma of, 142–44
    diagnosis of, 139–42, 156–57, 214,
        218
    dissociation by, 139, 148, 149,
        156–58, 164–65, 195–99, 223–27,
        231
    Gordon ego state of, 144, 145, 146,
        148, 150, 151–53, 157, 158
    as housepainter, 142, 145–46
    hypnosis used for, 224–25, 228
    James ego state of, 144, 145, 146,
        150, 157, 158, 225–26
    mother of, 143, 226–27
    recovery by, 223–27
    Uncle Dean as tormentor of,
        143–44, 152, 223–25
    Willie ego state of, 146, 149, 150,
        157, 158
genocide, 63
Grand Hotel Oloffson, 118–19
grandiose delusions, 185
Grass, Günter, 10
grief, 95, 148–49, 234
guilt, 178

Habitat for Humanity, 145, 226
habit strength, 20
"habitual dissociative reactions,"
    218–19
Haiti, 118–22
Harvard Medical School, 135
Harvard University, 64
heart failure, 10–11, 149

heights, fear of, 124–27, 128, 162,
    219
helplessness, 53
"hero missions," 179–83
hippocampus, 17, 18, 76
"holding environment," 71
Holmes, Oliver Wendell, 67
Holocaust, 63–66
homicide, 141
hominids, 49–50
hospitals, psychiatric, 9, 135–39
humanity, survival of, 49–50, 127–28,
    139, 232–33
humor, sense of, 5, 24, 105, 166–67,
    234
hunger, chronic, 63, 64
hypnosis:
    ambience for, 67–68
    dissociation and, 69–70, 71, 91–103
    examples of, 25, 43, 67–103,
        224–25, 228
    history of, 68–71
    memories recovered in, 70, 71,
        73–77, 228–29
    process of, 71–73, 77–103
    relaxation in, 78–80
    self-, 197
    trance induced by, 27, 68–73,
        77–80, 92–94, 113–14, 228–29
hysteria, 68, 70, 139–40, 154

iatrogenic effects, 140–41
illness, physical, 36, 51–52, 118,
    121–22, 186, 210–11
imagination, 7, 9, 73, 197
impersonation, 197
injuries, 129
insight meditation, 229
insomnia, 36, 64–66, 118, 125
insulin, 147
International Federation of Red
    Cross and Red Crescent Soci-
    eties, 63
introspection, 109

Janet, Pierre, 70
jealousy, 170–72, 195
Jimmie G. (case study), 210–11
journals, 228
Joyce, James, 114
Julia (case study), 21–26, 67–103
    Amelia ego state of, 91–94, 97–103,
        139
    appendectomy of, 41–42, 220
    background of, 21–26
    childhood trauma of, 23–26, 29–30,
        62, 80–103, 107–8, 230
    dissociation by, 25–26, 29–30,
        32–35, 41–42, 50–51, 91–103,
        104, 107–8, 113, 127, 146, 149,
        220, 231
    fugue of, 32–35
    hypnosis used for, 25, 43, 67–103,
        228
    Kate ego state of, 97–103, 127,
        139
    personality of, 21–22
    recovery by, 233–35
    repressed memories of, 80–103
    suicide attempt of, 22–23, 25, 30,
        233–34

Kenneth (case study), 124–27, 128,
    160, 162–64, 219, 242n
Korsakoff's syndrome, 210–11

language, 17–18, 19
Lars (case study), 187–88, 197, 217
La Salpêtrière, 70
Laura (case study), 123–24, 128, 160,
    220
legal issues, 140–41
lethargy, 123–24, 126, 128, 160,
    217
liars, pathological, 187–88, 195
life expectancy, 63
Lila (case study), 36, 41
limbic system, 19
"little coach" ritual, 89–90

Little Golden Books, 54
loneliness, 202, 203, 227, 234
Lorenz, Konrad, 201
Louis XVI, King of France, 68

McFarlane, Alexander, 52–53, 54
McLean Hospital, 135–39
Magda (case study), 64–66
magnetic trance, 68–69
mammillary bodies, 210–11
Marcie (case study), 10–11, 13–14
Marie Antoinette, Queen of France,
    68
marriage, 6–7, 40, 105–6, 109,
    110–12, 163–64, 168–77, 187–88
Mason (case study), 190–93, 197, 198,
    203–4
Matthew (case study), 55, 60–62,
    105–13, 117, 160–61, 218,
    229–30
meaning systems, 52–55, 62, 210–11,
    214
media, mass, 140–41
meditation, 229
Melody D. (case study), 201–2,
    217–18
memories:
    cognitive, 25
    declarative (explicit), 76
    false, 73–77
    lapses in, 109, 116–17, 131, 172–73,
        194–95, 216–17
    metaphor and, 73–74, 143–44
    neurological basis of, 76
    recovery of, 9, 43, 70, 71, 73–77,
        85–88, 103, 111–13, 225, 228–
        31
    research on, 75
    sensory, 230–31
    suppression of, 23–24, 29–30, 74,
        75, 80–103
    trauma and, 3–4, 17–18, 232–33
"memory work," 228
Meng (case study), 190–91, 218

Mesmer, Franz Anton, 68–69
metaphor, 73–74, 143–44
mimicry, 197
misanthropy, 125–26, 128
Mischel, Walter, 162, 241*n*
"mode," 7
moodiness, 162–63, 193–94
moral values, 211–12
mothers, 209–10
movies, 26–27, 113–14, 196, 218
Mozart, Wolfgang Amadeus, 69
multiple personality disorder, *see* dis-
    sociative identity disorder
Murdoch, Iris, 47
myopia, 147

narcissism, 208
Nathan (case study), 166–67, 193,
    196, 198, 216–17, 218
National Child Abuse and Neglect
    Data System (NCANDS), 238*n*
National Committee to Prevent Child
    Abuse, 51
National Institute of Mental Health,
    141–42
near-death experience, 11, 23
near-miss reaction, 114–15, 117
"nervous sleep," 69
neurohormones, 17
neurology, 17–18, 76, 147–48
neuropeptides, 76
neuroses, 70, 104
neurotransmitters, 76
New York Review of Books, 21
Nigeria, 177–79
nightmares, 64–66, 109, 147
non compos mentis, 156
norepinephrine, 17
Nørretranders, Tor, 102
nostalgia, 54

observing ego, 127–28, 130–31, 150,
    163, 165, 194, 218, 220–21,
    231–32

ocean imagery, 37–38, 39, 40, 41, 220,
    235
"one-pointed" concentration, 229

pain, 28, 38–39, 41–42, 59–60, 69, 95,
    109–10, 147, 176–77, 216–17,
    220
panic attacks, 109
Paracelsus, 140, 240*n*
paranoia, 19, 125–26, 128, 160, 162,
    185, 203
parasympathetic arrest, 149
Parker (case study), 209–10
pathological liars, 187–88, 195
perceptual field, 50
performance anxiety, 115–17, 218
persecution complex, 185
personality:
    assessment of, 161–64
    compartmentalization of, 100–101,
        166–68, 207–9
    definition of, 101, 208–9
    demarcation of, 155–56, 210–11, 219
    fragmentation of, *see* ego states
    protector, 151–53
    see also behavior
Personality and Assessment (Mischel),
    162
"phasing out," 218
possession, spirit, 153–54, 155
post-traumatic stress disorder, 4, 52,
    74, 76, 147
poverty, 63, 119–20
predators, 50
projective devices, 195
pseudoseizures, 147
psychoanalysis, 70
psychosis, 140–41
psychosomatic symptoms, 42, 202–3

rape, 13
rationalizations, 161, 216
reality:
    adaptation to, 175–77, 193

definition of, 159–60
detachment from, 37, 159–60,
    206–7, 214–15, 240n
immediate, 47–49
perception of, 30–31, 37–38, 52–55,
    62
present, 3, 149
regression, 186–87, 204, 218
rejection, social, 109, 125–26, 163
relationships, 215–17, 221–22
resiliencey, mental, 50–51
responsibility, personal, 109, 110,
    140–41, 155–58, 189–90, 204–14,
    215, 222, 230
reverie, 127
Richter, C. P., 149, 241n

Sacks, Oliver, 210–11
safety, sense of, 10, 179–84, 227–28,
    231
samadhi, 229
sanity, reclaimed, 214–15, 222, 223–35
Santayana, George, 192
Sarah (case study), 188–90, 198, 217
Satan, 154, 185
schizophrenia, 13, 148, 185
Schreiber, Flora Rheta, 196, 197
self:
    departures from, 19–20, 72, 116–17,
        214–15, 218, 220–21, 240n
    protection of, 151–53, 212–13
self-awareness, 3–14, 19–10, 21, 34–35
self-destructive behavior, 4, 9–10, 137
self-hypnosis, 197
self-identity, 240n
self-mutilation, 9–10, 137
self-pity, 213–14
"session rooms," 95
Seth (case study), 37–41, 220
sexuality, infantile, 74
shamantha, 229
shame, 95, 150
shin pan, 38–39, 42, 229
"silent witnessing," 229

Sizemore, Chris Costner, 197
sleep deprivation, 36, 64–66, 118, 125
sleepiness, 123–24, 128, 160, 217
social workers, 179
sociopathy, 185, 208
solar plexus, 39
soul, 40, 208–14
"spaciness," 19–20, 105–13, 147,
    160–61, 194–95, 218–19
startle responses, 147
starvation, 10–11
stereotypes, female, 204
stress:
    combat, 28, 31–32, 70, 76
    dissociation triggered by, 35–36
    physical response to, 17–18, 185
    post-traumatic, 4, 52, 74, 76, 147
    protracted, 149, 208
suffering, 20–21, 109–10, 227
suggestibility, 73–77
suicide, 4, 5, 11–12, 22–23, 25, 30,
    109, 144–45, 147, 150, 175,
    188–90, 217, 223–25, 233–34
supervisory attention, 77
surgery, 58–60
survival mechanisms, 49–51
Sybil (Schreiber), 196, 197
symbolism, 31–32

Tale of Two Cities, A (Dickens), 176
Taoism, 229
thalamus, 17
therapy:
    family, 179
    necessity of, 23, 108–9, 111, 112,
        189–90
    progress in, 108–9, 111, 112,
        189–90, 223–27, 233–35
thiamine deficiency, 210–11
Thich Nhat Hanh, 229
Three Faces of Eve, The, 196, 197
Tin Drum, The, 10
trance, 27, 68–73, 77–80, 92–94,
    113–14, 228–29

trauma:
  brain function and, 17–18, 19, 20,
    76, 147–48, 210–11, 223
  chronic, 20, 117, 141
  definition of, 52–53
  flashbacks and, 17–20, 31–32,
    117–23, 147, 225
  memory and, 3–4, 17–18, 232–33
  primary, 55–62
  psychological impact of, 52–62
  recovery from, 15–17, 20–21, 227–35
  reenactment of, 201–2
  secondary, 62–66, 104
  self-awareness and, 3–14, 19–20, 21,
    34–35
  survival after, 5–6, 47–66, 100–101,
    108, 144, 148–49, 173, 175–77,
    189–90, 203, 211–13, 227,
    230–35
  view of reality changed by, 52–55,
    62
trauma-related dissociative episodes,
  see ego states
truth, historical versus narrative, 76–77
"tune-ups," 233
turtles, 50, 232
Twain, Mark, 222

unconsciousness, 74

Valium, 204
van der Kolk, Bessel A., 201–2
vengeance, 232
victimization, 183–84, 212–14, 230
Vietnam War, 183–84, 191–92,
  202
vigilantism, 179–83
violence:
  dissociation and, 183–86
  domestic, 51, 60–62, 187–88
  social, 51, 179–83, 184
  sources of, 184–85, 216, 227–28
vipasana, 229
visual acuity, 147
voices, internal, 157–58, 217, 223–25
voodoo, 10, 119–21, 122

war, 28, 31–32, 63, 64, 66, 70, 76,
  183–84, 190–92, 238n–39n
weapons, 10, 179–84
weddings, 116–17
Welty, Eudora, 159
Woodward, Joanne, 196
World Disaster Report, 63
World Health Organization,
  63
World War II, 66, 70, 238n–39n

yi-ping, 154